A COLOR ATLAS OF ENDOVASCULAR SURGERY

A COLOR ATLAS OF ENDOVASCULAR SURGERY

Interventional techniques in vascular disease

Rodney A. White
Chief of Vascular Surgery
Harbor-UCLA Medical Center
and
Associate Professor of Surgery
UCLA School of Medicine
California, USA

Geoffrey H. White
Vascular Surgeon
University of Sydney and
The Royal Prince Alfred Hospital
Sydney, Australia

J. B. LIPPINCOTT COMPANY *Philadelphia*
New York   St. Louis   San Francisco

First edition 1990

© 1990 Chapman and Hall

Distributed in the USA and Canada
by J. B. Lippincott Company,
East Washington Square,
Philadelphia, PA 19105, USA
Printed and bound in Hong Kong

ISBN 0-397-58328-1

Library of Congress Catalog Card
Number is available.

Contents

Preface

Cardiovascular disease is the leading cause of death in most countries which have a high socioeconomic status. In the United States alone it was estimated in 1986 that approximately 57 million people were afflicted with atherosclerotic cardiovascular disorders; 43 million of those were under the age of 65, with 10 million being symptomatic. There were an estimated 768 000 coronary deaths and 50 000 fatalities related to peripheral vascular disease. Approximately 1 million interventions are performed each year in the United States for vascular illnesses, with cardiac disease being approximately 60% of this volume.

In light of the fact that we are currently treating occlusive vascular disease using methods which have limited benefit in the majority of symptomatic patients, there is a significant interest in improving our knowledge of the aetiology of atherosclerosis as a means of enhancing diagnosis and therapy. Prophylaxis is obviously the best approach, but at present a significant percentage of the population has advanced disease. An increasing mean age of the population substantiates the need to improve methods of bypassing or disobliterating occluded vessels.

Newer interventional methods to recanalize stenotic and occluded vascular segments, including instruments such as atherectomy devices, lasers, ultrasound ablators and stents, are being evaluated in conjunction with more conventional techniques such as balloon dilatation, thrombolysis and surgical intervention. The devices are being evaluated by the more precise intravascular imaging techniques of angioscopy and computerized ultrasound.

This book reviews the knowledge of the aetiology, natural history and quantitation of atherosclerosis, and details the current status and utility of endovascular surgical devices and procedures. This topic is particularly well suited for presentation in an atlas format, since much of the technology is best described by illustrations of the devices, angiograms, angioscopic images, histological specimens, etc. Figures are described by brief captions and accompanying text, with pertinent statements regarding current advantages, limitations and perspectives for future development. Key references are also cited to provide further documentation for points of particular interest, and to establish a bibliography covering controversial points.

Acknowledgements

We would like to especially recognize the assistance and support of George Kopchok, Biomedical Engineer at the Vascular Research Laboratory, Harbor-UCLA Medical Center, for his role in many of the procedures and in producing illustrative material. We would also like to thank Gloria Stevens for her untiring and conscientious efforts in word processing the manuscript material, and for her organizational skills.

We wish to acknowledge the invaluable support of Chapman and Hall in the preparation and timely completion of this book. In particular, we thank Helen Hadjidimitriadou, Medical Editor, for her outstanding effort which enabled rapid and accurate publication. Her tireless work was beyond our expectations. We thank Mick Brennan, independent design consultant, for his expert arrangement of the text and illustrations. We are also indebted to Dr Peter Altman, Medical Publisher, for initiating the development of this text and for his support throughout the endeavour.

Once more, our wives and families have been very understanding and supportive during the time spent in preparing the manuscript, and this book is dedicated to them.

Rodney A. White
Geoffrey H. White
June 1990

1 The Atherosclerotic Lesion

PATHOGENESIS OF ATHEROSCLEROSIS

Atherosclerosis is primarily an intimal disease, with secondary changes subsequently occurring in the media of the artery. The three main constituents of an early lesion are smooth muscle cells, extracellular matrix (collagen, elastin and proteoglycan), and lipid. These early or 'simple' plaques progress to complex lesions, with accumulation of cellular debris, haemorrhage and calcification of non-viable components.

A schematic account of the contemporary theory regarding the development of the atherosclerotic lesion is illustrated in Fig. 1.1. Figs. 1.2 and 1.3 demonstrate experimental findings which support the concept proposed in Fig. 1.1. Theories concerning the aetiologies for the development of atherosclerotic lesions are illustrated in the following discussion.

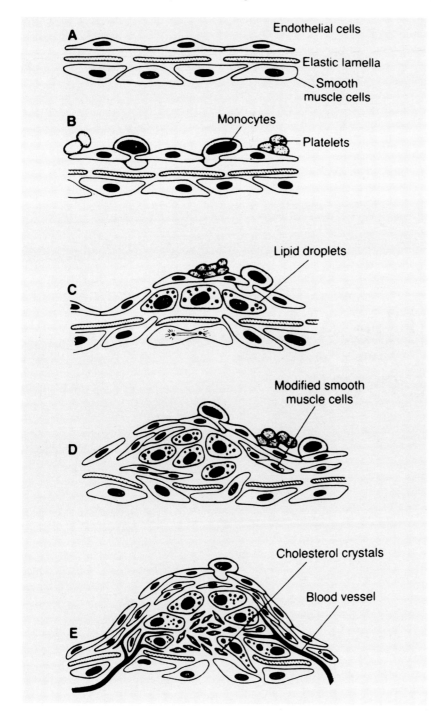

Fig. 1.1 Postulated sequence of events in the pathogenesis of atherosclerosis. (a) Normal vessel wall. **(b)** Subtle endothelial injury leads to attachment of monocytes and platelets. **(c)** Monocytes infiltrate the intima and accumulate lipid. Smooth muscle cells proliferate in response to growth factors secreted by platelets, endothelium and macrophages. **(d)** Smooth muscle cells migrate into the subendothelial space, and some of them accumulate lipid droplets. **(e)** Foam cell population, consisting of lipid-containing macrophages and smooth muscle cells, continues to build up. Additional lipid accumulates extracellularly as cholesterol crystals. (From Buja, 1987, with permission.)

Theory 1: response to injury

The original concept of response to injury is illustrated in Fig. 1.4; this was presented by Ross and Harker in 1976. The revised model of this theory was presented in 1986, and is depicted in Fig. 1.5.

According to the original hypothesis, two different cyclic events may occur (Fig. 1.4): the

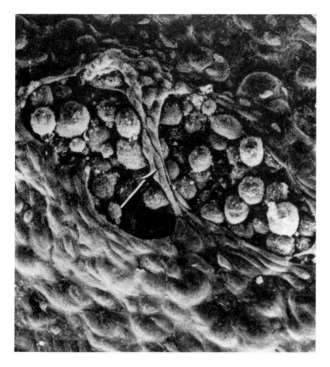

Fig. 1.2 Surface of a fatty streak in a pigtail monkey. The endothelium has retracted over a portion of the lesion, exposing underlying lipid-laden macrophages. A bridge of endothelial cells (arrow) is present over the centre of the region of exposed macrophages. Such areas of endothelial retraction were commonly observed over fatty streaks in the iliac arteries, after five months of induced hypercholesterolaemia in monkeys. SEM, ×600. (From Ross, 1986, with permission.)

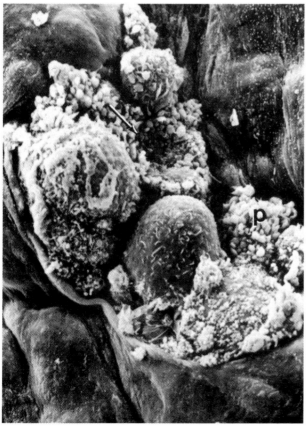

Fig. 1.3 Small segment of a fatty streak in a pigtail monkey. The endothelial cover has presumably been lost through endothelial retraction, exposing several underlying macrophages. At one site (arrow) a small platelet thrombus has formed in a crater-like region. This area may have previously been the site of a macrophage. Platelets (p) are attached to exposed macrophages and subendothelial connective tissue (not shown). These changes occur at sites which one to two months later are involved with proliferative fibrous plaques containing smooth muscle cells. SEM ×7000. (From Ross, 1986, with permission.)

outer, or regression cycle may represent common single occurrences in all individuals in which endothelial injury leads to desquamation, platelet adherence, aggregation and release. This is followed by intimal smooth muscle proliferation and connective tissue formation. If the injury is a single event, the lesions may go on to heal and thus regression occurs.

The inner, or progression cycle demonstrates the possible consequences of repeated or chronic endothelial injury as may result from chronic hyperlipidaemia. In this instance, lipid deposition as well as continued smooth muscle proliferation may occur after recurrent sequences of proliferation and regression, leading to complicated lesions which calcify. These lesions go on to pro-

duce clinical sequelae such as thrombosis and infarction.

According to the revised hypothesis (Fig. 1.5), advanced intimal proliferative lesions of atherosclerosis may occur by at least two pathways. The pathway demonstrated by the clockwise (long) arrows to the right has been observed in experimentally induced hypercholesterolaemia. Injury to the endothelium (A) may induce growth factor secretion (short arrow). Monocytes attach to endothelium (B) which may continue to secrete growth factors (short arrow). Subendothelial migration of monocytes (C) may lead to fatty streak formation and release of growth factors such as PDGF (short arrow). Fatty streaks may become directly converted to fibrous plaques

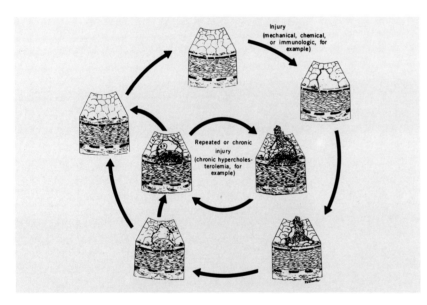

Fig. 1.4 Response to injury theory. A schematic summary of the hypothesis that two different cyclic events may be involved in the pathogenesis of atherosclerosis. (From Ross and Harker, 1976, with permission.)

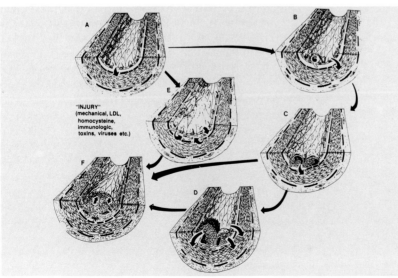

Fig. 1.5 Revised response to injury theory. A schematic summary of the hypothesis that intimal proliferative lesions of atherosclerosis may occur by at least two pathways. (From Ross, 1986, with permission.)

(long arrow C-F), through release of growth factors from macrophages, endothelial cells, or both. Macrophages may also stimulate or injure the overlying endothelium. In some cases, they may lose their endothelial cover and platelet attachment may occur (D), providing three possible sources of growth factors – platelets, macrophages and endothelium (short arrows). Some of the smooth muscle cells in the proliferative lesion itself (F) may form and secrete growth factors such as PDGF (short arrows).

An alternative pathway to the development of advanced atherosclerotic lesions is shown by the arrows from A to E to F. In this case, the endothelium may be injured but remains intact. Increased endothelial turnover may result in growth factor formation by endothelial cells (A). This may stimulate migration of smooth muscle cells from the media to the intima, accompanied by endogenous production of PDGF by smooth muscle as well as growth factor secretion from the 'injured' endothelial cells (E). These interactions could then lead to fibrous plaque formation and further progression of the lesion (F).

The multiple sources and complex interactions of smooth muscle cell stimulation by growth factors from platelets, monocytes and macrophages, endothelial cells etc. lead to a continuous lesion development, if the injury pattern persists (Figs 1.6 and 1.7).

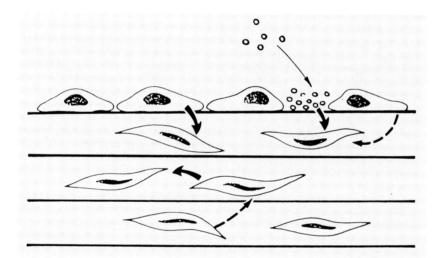

Fig. 1.6 Sources of smooth muscle cell stimulation. A schematic representation of an artery in cross-section, showing possible sources of growth promoting (heavy arrows) and growth inhibiting (broken arrows) activity for smooth muscle cells. Endothelial cells and platelets adhering to denuded regions, as well as medial smooth muscle cells, can release growth factors; endothelial and medial smooth muscle cells can release heparin-like growth inhibitors. (From Clowes, 1989, with permission.)

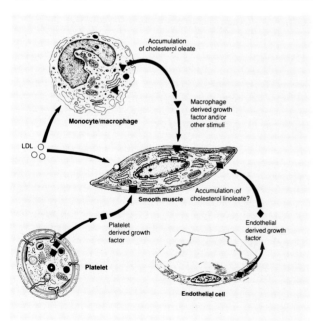

Fig. 1.7 Susceptibility of smooth muscle cells. A schematic representation of the proposal that smooth muscle cells are susceptible to at least four potentially stimulatory growth factors: platelet-derived (PDGF), endothelial-derived (EDGF), monocyte/macrophage-derived (MDGF) and LDL. The particular importance of each of these growth factors, as a cause of smooth muscle proliferation in the genesis of atherosclerotic lesions, needs to be better defined for each special set of circumstances. These investigations provide important opportunities for further research. (From Ross, 1981, with permission.)

Theory 2: lipid accumulation

This theory focuses on hyperlipidaemia as the cause of the primary lesion. The accumulation of lipids also corresponds to the contemporary theory that control of serum lipids is an impor- tant factor in not only limiting the development of atherosclerotic lesions, but also in helping to control the progression of disease (Figs 1.8, 1.9 and 1.10).

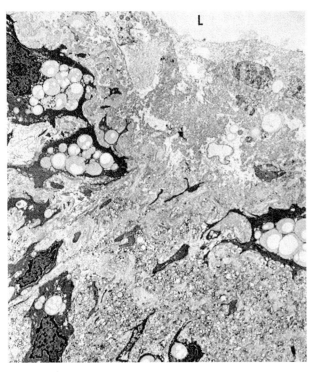

Fig. 1.8 Portion of an intimal lesion in the iliac artery of a monkey. This monkey was on a hyperlipidaemic diet for six months following balloon injury. Most of the smooth muscle cells in the lesion contain large lipid deposits. The cells are surrounded by small, globular, membranous deposits in the connective tissue. An endothelial cover is lacking on the luminal surface (L), at the crest of the lesion. (From Ross and Harker, 1976, with permission, Copyright 1976 by the AAAS.)

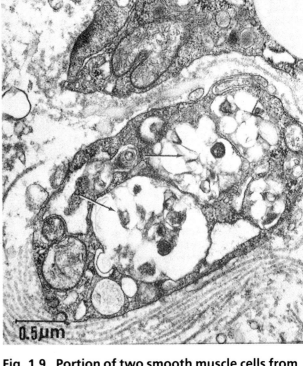

Fig. 1.9 Portion of two smooth muscle cells from a 9-month lesion in a monkey with chronic hyperlipidaemia. The cells are surrounded by numerous collagen fibrils. In one of the cells, secondary lysosomes (arrow) are visible; they contain membranous globules or deposits which represent a breakdown of the large, amorphous lipid droplets (see cell on the upper right). The breakdown products are similar in appearance to the membranous deposits seen in the extracellular space surrounding these two cells. (From Ross and Harker, 1976, with permission.)

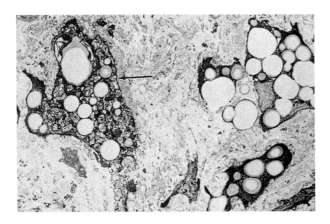

Fig. 1.10 Lesion from a chronically hyperlipidaemic monkey. The plasma membrane of the smooth muscle cell on the left is broken (arrow), demonstrating that the cell has undergone necrosis and is in the process of releasing its lipid inclusions into the extracellular compartment. Several other intact, lipid-laden smooth muscle cells are also visible. (From Ross and Harker, 1976, with permission.)

Theory 3: monoclonal lesions

According to this theory, stimulation of single cells produces monoclonal lesions similar to neoplasms. This hypothesis implicates viruses or other carcinogens as aetiological agents in this process.

DEVELOPMENT OF ATHEROSCLEROTIC LESIONS

Fatty streaks

Many experts believe that the atherosclerotic process begins in childhood with the development of flat, lipid-rich intimal lesions. Histologically, the organization of lesions in the thickened intima resembles the structure of the media of the arterial wall (Figs 1.11 and 1.12).

Fibrous plaques

Progressive thickening of a simple lesion by continued proliferation of smooth muscle cells and production of extracellular matrix leads to stenotic or occlusive fibrous lesions, which first appear in human arteries at 25 years of age or over. There is debate as to whether these lesions represent the progression of fatty streaks (Figs 1.13 and 1.14).

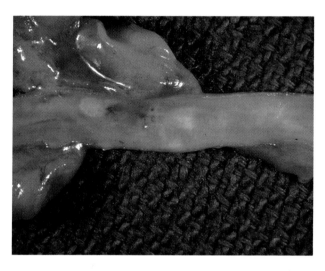

Fig. 1.11 Lipid-rich deposits in the renal artery of a 2-year-old child.

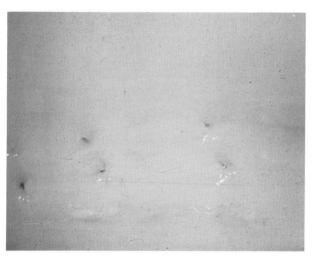

Fig. 1.12 Yellowish fatty streaks along the posterior surface of the aorta in a 14-year-old male.

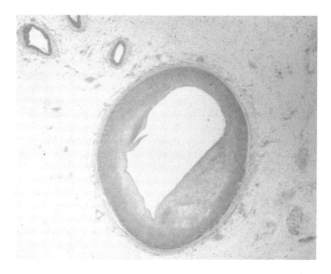

Fig. 1.13 Small fibrous lesion in the coronary artery. H&E, ×4.

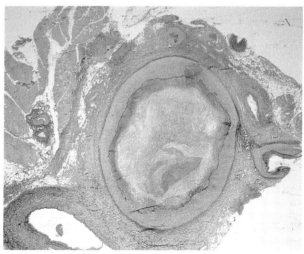

Fig. 1.14 Large fibrous occlusion of the femoral artery with thrombosis of the residual lumen. Verhoeff van Giessen, ×4.

Complex lesions

Complex atherosclerotic lesions develop in anoxic areas of the vessel wall by accumulation of cellular debris, haemorrhage and calcification. Stenotic lesions may lead to occlusion (Fig. 1.15), or luminal surfaces may ulcerate producing thrombogenic, potentially embolic surfaces (Fig. 1.16).

DISTRIBUTION OF ATHEROSCLEROSIS

Atherosclerosis initially occurs in low shear stress areas at the orifices of bifurcations of branch

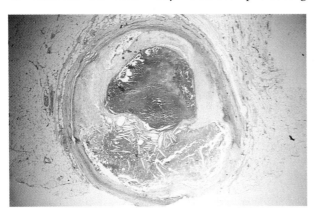

Fig. 1.15 Complex coronary artery atheroma. Calcification of non-viable components and concomitant thrombosis of the lumen occurs in complex lesions. H&E, ×4.

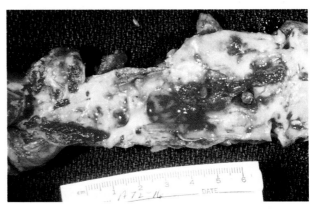

Fig. 1.16 Severely diseased abdominal aorta. Ulcerated complex lesions are seen.

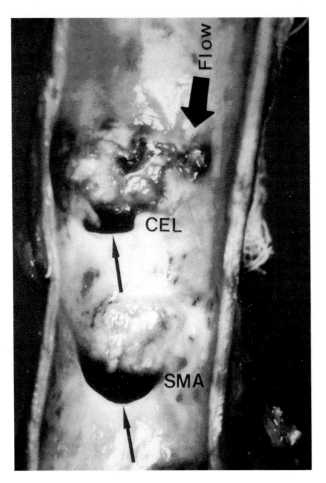

Fig. 1.17 Coeliac and superior mesenteric ostia of human aorta. Note the prominent plaque formation at the upstream rim of the ostia, with no plaque formation on the flow divider (arrows) which is exposed to high shear stress. CEL=coeliac artery; SMA = superior mesenteric artery. (From Zarins and Glagov, 1986, with permission.)

vessels, and at transition sites (Fig. 1.17). Approximately 70% of both coronary and peripheral lesions develop with an eccentric position in the vessel lumen, so that the residual lumen is usually 'off centre' in relation to the outside walls of the artery (Fig. 1.18). This eccentric position of lesions has important implications for interventional therapies such as endarterectomy, balloon angioplasty, etc.

Early stages of lesion development may be associated with over-compensation in the outside diameter of the vessel wall. However, when the degree of stenosis is greater than 40%, the plaque area continues to increase to involve the entire circumference of the vessel, whilst the artery no longer enlarges at a rate sufficient to prevent narrowing of the lumen (Figs 1.19 and 1.20).

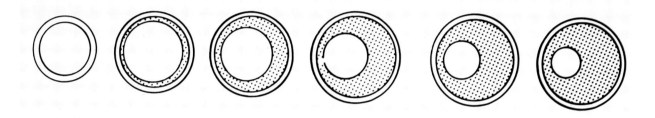

Fig. 1.18 Changes in atherosclerotic arteries. A diagrammatic representation of a possible sequence of changes that may eventually lead to lumen narrowing. The artery initially enlarges (from left to right) in association with plaque accumulation to maintain an adequate, if not a normal, lumen area. (Adapted from Glagov et al., 1987, with permission.)

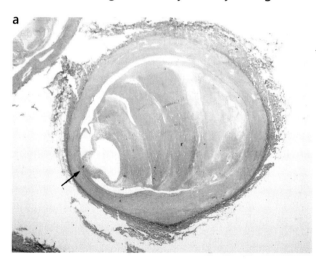

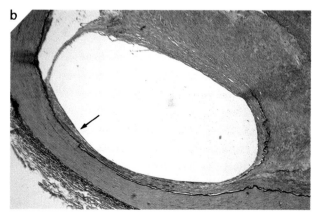

Fig. 1.19 Superficial femoral artery lesion with eccentric lumen. This resulted from sequential narrowing by laminated enlargement of the obstruction (a). LM, ×4. (b) A magnified view of the residual lumen is demonstrating a relatively normal wall architecture on one aspect (arrows), and the occlusive lesion on the opposite wall. Verhoeff van Giessen, × 40.

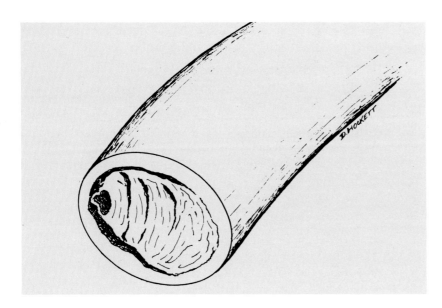

Fig. 1.20 Three-dimensional diagram of the lesion seen in Fig. 1.19. This three-dimensional display will be used in subsequent chapters to emphasize the importance of the eccentric distribution of lesions on the mechanisms of action, performance and limitation of current angioplasty devices and guidance methods.

References

Buja, L.M. (1987) The vascular system, in *Basic Pathology*, 4th edn. (eds S.L. Robbins and V. Kumar), Saunders, Philadelphia, pp. 285–320.

Clowes, A. (1989) Theories of atherosclerosis, in *Atherosclerosis and Arteriosclerosis: Human Pathology and Experimental Animal Methods and Models* (ed. R.A. White), CRC Press, Boca Raton, pp. 4–15.

Glagov, S., Weisenberg, E., Zarins, C. *et al.* (1987) Compensatory enlargement of human atherosclerotic coronary arteries. *New. Engl. J. Med.*, **316**, 1371–5.

Ross, R. (1981) Atherosclerosis: a problem of the biology of arterial wall cells and their interactions with blood components. *Atherosclerosis*, **1**, 293–311.

Ross, R. (1986) Patholgenesis of atherosclerosis—an update. *New Engl. J. Med.*, **314**, 488–500.

Ross, R. and Harker, L. (1976) Hyperlipidemia and atherosclerosis. *Science*, **193**, 1094–100.

Zarins, C.K. and Glagov, S. (1986) Pathophysiology of human atherosclerosis, in *Vascular Surgery: Principles and Practice* (eds S.E. Wilson *et al.*), McGraw-Hill, New York, p. 23.

2 Development of Interventional Methods in Relation to Lesion Distribution

The patterns of development of atherosclerotic lesions are integral to the design, application and success of various interventional methods. Conventional vascular reconstructions bypass heavily diseased or occluded arterial segments by connecting relatively normal areas in the vessel proximal and distal to the lesions (Fig. 2.1).

Endarterectomy relies on the eccentric (usually posterior), localized nature of lesions, so that complete removal can be accomplished through a transmural incision, removing the plaque with a smooth transition to the adjacent luminal surface (Fig. 2.2).

Successful balloon angioplasty relies on accomplishing a fracture of the arterial lesion, thus enlarging the lumen and displacing the pla-

que. Eccentric positioning of the atherosclerotic lesions within the artery wall predisposes to controlled fracture of the thinner portion of the plaque, displacing the majority of the mass to create a neolumen (Figs 2.3 and 2.4).

An additional factor which enhances the success rate of transluminal recanalizations over the expected outcome, as estimated from preintervention angiography, is that the atherosclerotic lesions are usually localized within one area of the arterial segment. Softer clot and organized material fill the lumen proximal to the lesion to the site of a patent branch artery, carrying collateral flow distally (Fig. 2.5).

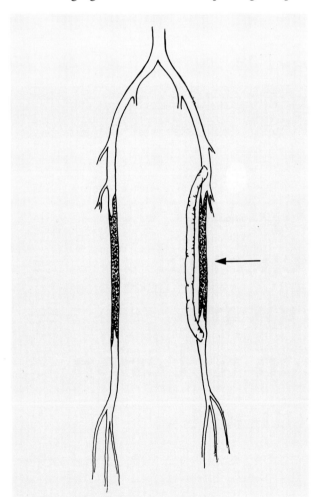

Fig. 2.1 Schematic representation of conventional vascular reconstruction. Occluded arterial segment (arrow).

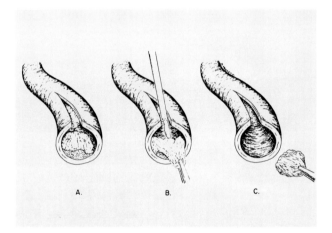

Fig. 2.2 Schematic representation of endarterectomy.

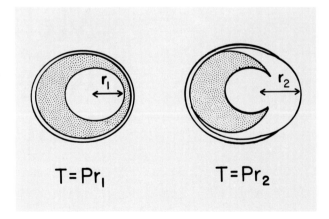

Fig. 2.3 Mechanism by which effective lumen radius is increased by balloon dilatation. A critical level of tangential tension (T) may be necessary to prevent collapse. (From Zarins and Glagov, 1986, with permission.)

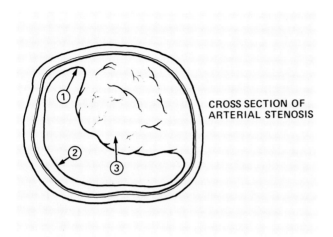

CROSS SECTION OF
ARTERIAL STENOSIS

Fig. 2.4 Mechanisms of vessel enlargement. 1 and **2** Disruption of the plaque artery junction produces 85–95% of the lumen enlargement. **3** It also produces plaque fluid extrusion (5–14%) and plaque compaction (<1%). (From Zimmerman and Fogarty, 1986, with permission.)

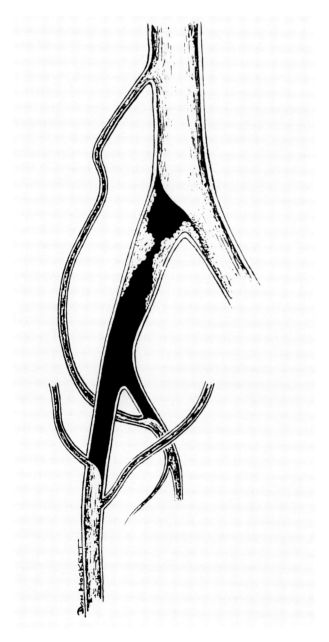

Fig. 2.5 Schematic representation of a short lesion in the iliac artery. There is propagation of clot and soft material (white-shaded area) proximal and distal to the atherosclerotic narrowing.

The majority of long occlusions, evident on angiography, have significant proportions of the segment obstructed by variable stages of organizing thrombus, as demonstrated. For this reason, the apparent length of many occlusions can be shortened by thrombolytic therapy. The residual atherosclerotic lesion can subsequently be treated by various interventional methods. The significant component of soft material also enables successful passage of wires across many long segment occlusions.

The success rate of current devices is enhanced by this factor, while failures are related to inadequate guidance and debulking of lesions in segments which are occluded by fibrotic or calcified material.

References

Zarins, C. and Glagov, S. (1986) Morphologic alterations after transluminal angioplasty, in *Vascular Surgery: Principles and Practice* (eds S.E. Wilson *et al.*), McGraw-Hill, New York, pp. 288–96.

Zimmerman, J.H. and Fogarty, T.J. (1986) Adjunctive intraoperative dilatation (angioplasty), in *Vascular Surgery: Principles and Practices* (eds S.E. Wilson *et al.*), McGraw-Hill, New York, pp. 297–302.

3 Intraluminal Access Techniques

PERCUTANEOUS VASCULAR ACCESS

Percutaneous vascular access is usually obtained by the Seldinger technique (Block, 1984). A bevelled needle is introduced through the arterial wall, after careful palpation of the arterial pulse. Usually, a small skin incision is made with a scalpel blade, to facilitate subsequent insertion of vessel dilators and instruments. The needle is slowly withdrawn until the return of arterial blood is achieved, signifying that the needle tip is positioned in the arterial lumen. A guidewire is then introduced through the central lumen of the needle, and is positioned under fluoroscopic control.

For many procedures, an introducer sheath is threaded over the guidewire after passage of a vascular dilator. The sheath diameter is determined by the size of the balloon or instrument which is to be passed through the sheath lumen into the vessel.

Percutaneous access via the femoral artery

Access for many percutaneous procedures is obtained by cannulation of the common femoral artery. The aortic bifurcation and iliac arteries are most effectively approached by an ipsilateral retrograde puncture of the femoral artery (Fig. 3.1a–e); lesions of the infrainguinal vessels are approached via an ipsilateral antegrade femoral artery puncture (Fig. 3.2a–f). This technique is more difficult because of the rapid decrease in diameter from the common femoral to superficial femoral arteries, and also due to the prominence of the lower abdominal wall and inguinal fat fold in many patients.

Lesions close to the usual femoral puncture site require careful consideration in order to assess the best route. A contralateral approach may often be preferred for treatment of lesions to the distal external iliac, common femoral and profunda arteries. Alternatively, the femoral puncture may be made more proximal or distal than usual, to accommodate access to selected lesions in this region.

Alternative entry approaches include the axillary, brachial and superficial femoral arteries, and rarely the popliteal artery. There are occasional indications for direct puncture of bypass grafts, either in the subcutaneous plane or deep in muscle groups. Puncture of the external iliac artery above the inguinal ligament may facilitate antegrade access to the femoral vessels, but it caries a higher risk of serious haemorrhage because of leakage into the retroperitoneum.

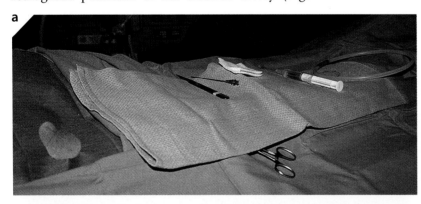

a

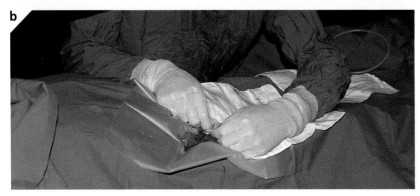

b

Fig. 3.1a Retrograde approach. Transfemoral angiography of the aorta for examination of the run-off vessels for coronary angiography, and for angioplasty of the iliac arteries or proximal vessels, is usually performed by retrograde percutaneous cannulation of the common femoral artery. Access to this vesssel is achieved by preparing a sterile field over the femoral vessels.

Fig. 3.1b Retrograde approach. A winged-tip needle is shown after introduction into the right femoral artery. Transmission of the arterial pulse to the needle is a useful indicator that the artery has been penetrated.

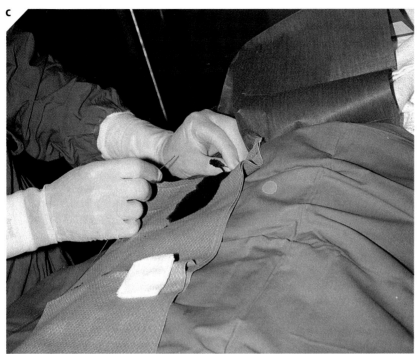

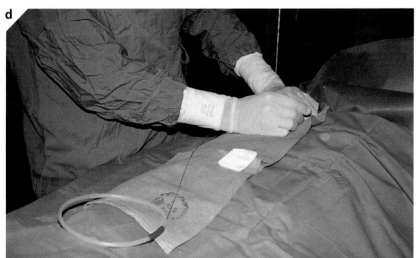

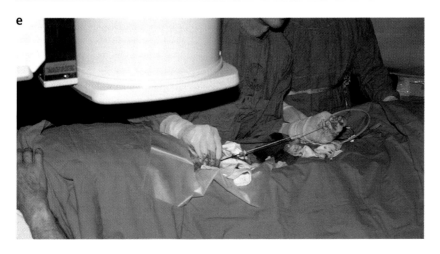

Fig. 3.1c Retrograde approach. The stylet is removed from the needle, and the needle is gently retracted until a spurt of arterial blood indicates successful positioning of the needle tip within the lumen of the vessel. Poor blood flow from the needle indicates that the tip is misplaced or is too close to the arterial wall; in this case, guidewire passage carries a high risk of wall dissection.

Fig. 3.1d Retrograde approach. The needle is now carefully held in this position while the guidewire is introduced. A short guidance cannula facilitates entry of the guidewire into the needle. Progress of the guidewire along the arterial lumen should be monitored by fluoroscopy, to avoid diversion into arterial branches or dissection of the vessel wall. Resistance to passage indicates possible misdirection or wall trauma.

Fig. 3.1e Retrograde approach. Once the guidewire has been satisfactorily positioned, a vessel dilator and introducing sheath may be advanced simul- taneously over the guidewire, with the dilator preceding the sheath by several inches. Commonly used sheaths have an attached sidearm which may be used for injection of radiological contrast dyes, anticoagulation agents or other solutions. Following introduction, the guidewire and dilator are removed from the sheath. A haemostatic valve prevents excessive blood loss, although minor leakage around the guidewires or instruments is common. Most angioplasty instruments are introduced via the sheath over the guidewire, for safer manipulation within the lumen.

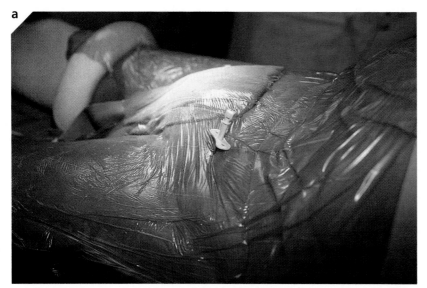

Fig. 3.2a Antegrade needle insertion into the left femoral artery. This approach provides access to vessels downstream from the femoral insertion site (femoral, popliteal and tibial arteries). The angle of insertion tends to direct guidewires into the profunda femoris artery. Some recently developed needles have side-facing distal openings near the tip, to facilitate antegrade or angulated entry of the guidewire into the lumen.

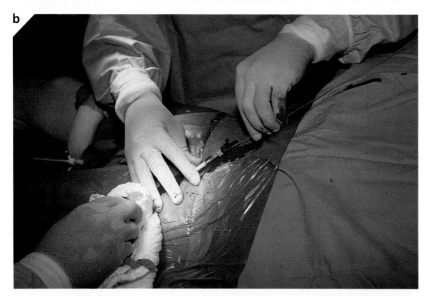

Fig. 3.2b Antegrade approach. The guidewire is being introduced with the needle held at a shallow angle to the cannulated artery, to direct it into the superficial femoral artery rather than the profunda system.

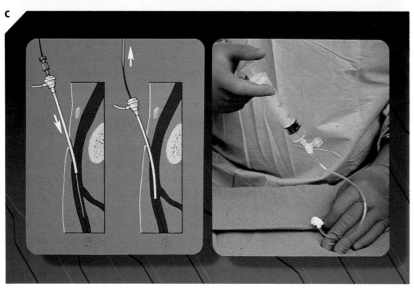

Fig. 3.2c Antegrade approach. Diagrammatic representation of a sheath (white) over the dilator (blue) which has been tracked over the guidewire. Injection of contrast medium via the sidearm is used to confirm positioning.

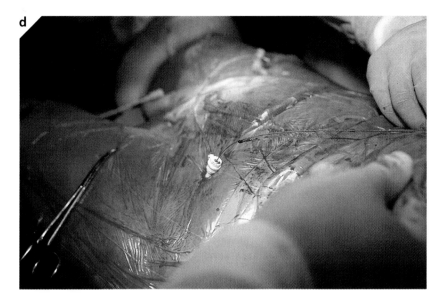

Fig. 3.2d Antegrade approach.
An 8F sheath, with sidearm injection port and haemostatic valve hub, has been inserted over the guidewire. In this case, a laser thermal probe of 2.5 mm diameter is threaded via the sheath, over the guidewire.

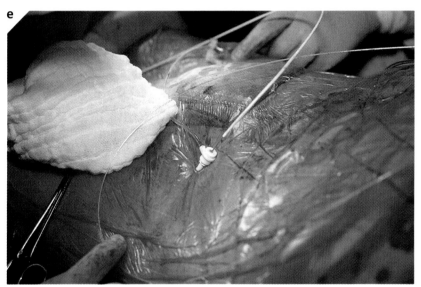

Fig. 3.2e Antegrade approach.
An angioscope of 2.3 mm diameter is inserted percutaneously via the sheath, to monitor the effects of the laser probe on the vessel wall. The angioscope may be inserted over the guidewire or independently.

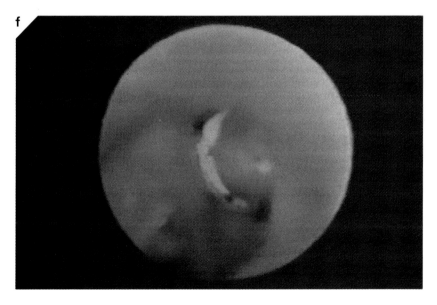

Fig. 3.2f Antegrade approach.
Angioscopic image of a guidewire passing into an arterial branch from the central lumen.

INTRAOPERATIVE ARTERIAL ACCESS

Intraoperative exposure and access to the femoral artery is commonly gained by longitudinal skin incision and sharp dissection (Fig. 3.3a–c). Atraumatic clamps are applied to the common femoral, superficial femoral and profunda femoris arteries, and to any minor branches in the field (see Fig. 3.3a). The arteriotomy incision may be longitudinal or transverse. The vascular clamps assure a bloodless field.

Angioplasty devices and other instruments may then be inserted directly into the opened vessel (see Fig. 3.3b). The vessel wall and entry site can be protected by a sheath similar to those used for percutaneous access (see Fig. 3.3c).

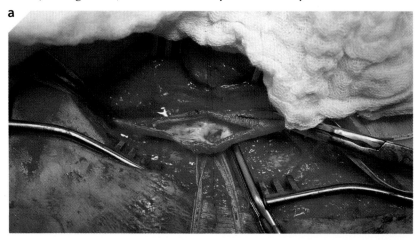

Fig. 3.3a Intraoperative arterial access. Atraumatic clamps are applied to the femoral, superficial and profunda femoris arteries as well as to minor branches.

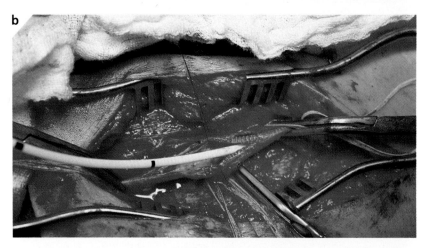

Fig. 3.3b Intraoperative arterial access. The occluded limb of an aorta-bifemoral bypass graft is being cannulated from the femoral approach.

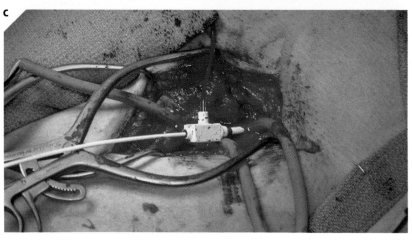

Fig. 3.3c Intraoperative arterial access. A Teflon loop around the artery holds the sheath in place and prevents blood loss.

Newer intraoperative and percutaneous devices are being developed, to decrease the trauma associated with repeated instrument introduction, to provide better haemostasis and to facilitate removal of intraluminal material. The Fogarty Expandable Access Device (Fig. 3.4) belongs to this category. This consists of an expandable tube which can be reduced in diameter by advancing a stylet that passes through a hub at its proximal end.

The purpose of the Expandable Access Device is to provide a flexible lining through which various instruments can be passed. This concept has the following characteristics:

1   The device can be introduced through a puncture or cut-down, in a low profile configuration; once in position, it can be expanded to the size of the vessel, providing control of antegrade and collateral blood flow.

2   Its flexible nature allows it to conform to the anatomy of the vessel and site of entry.

3   It has the ability to expand inside the vessel puncture, and also to contract around captured material to remove it from the vessel.

These characteristics suggest several potential clinical advantages in using this type of device for percutaneous and intraoperative procedures:

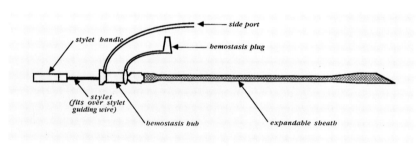

Fig. 3.4 Fogarty Expandable Sheath. Diagrammatic representation.

(a)   Due to its low profile and flexibility, the sheath can be placed to more distal locations, thus projecting the entire length of the vessel as opposed to the arteriotomy or puncture site alone. This lining conduit facilitates rapid placement of various instruments, with limited need for radiographic guidance.

(b)   Material can be 'funnelled' into the expandable lumen, facilitating its retrieval.

(c)   The lumen can act as a flexible mouth, to retain retrieved material and facilitate its removal from the vessel.

(d)   Occlusive material, too large to be managed with a percutaneous procedure, may be trapped in the distal end of the expandable lumen and morcelated into more manageable sections.

(e)   Morcelation of trapped material may be accomplished with less risk of injury to the vessel wall, as the sheath shields the vessel wall from the morcelating instrument.

(f)   Collateral blood flow can be occluded by expansion of lumen, allowing clearer views to be obtained during angioscopy. A reduction in flush volume may also be noted during angioscopy.

(g)   A new 'iris'-type haemostatic valve allows removal of the thrombus directly through the expansion sheath (Fig. 3.5)

The adjustable haemostatic, self-closing valve has been designed to be used in percutaneous as well as intraoperative procedures. The unique 'iris'-type valve (Fig. 3.6a) offers the following benefits:

1 An adjustable central lumen with a self-closing feature (Fig. 3.6b).

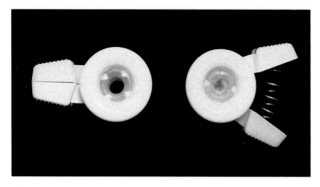

2 Single hand operation with atraumatic soft seal in sizes 0–9F or 0–15F.

3 Simultaneous atraumatic sealing around the catheter and adjacent guidewire.

4 Available in various configurations: side port, standard luer fittings.

Fig. 3.5 Expandable Access Device. This is fitted with the iris haemostatic valve.

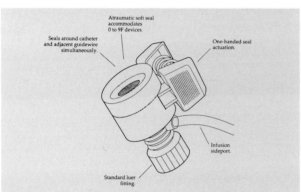

Fig. 3.6a 'Iris'-type valve. Diagrammatic representation.

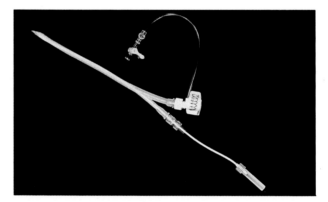

Fig. 3.6b 'Iris'-type valve. It features an adjustable central lumen which is self-closing.

References

Montarjeme, A. (1989) Thrombolytic therapy in arterial occlusion and graft thrombosis. *Semin. Vasc. Surg.* **2**, 155–78.

4 Balloon Angioplasty

Coauthored by
Dr Richard Waugh
Department of Radiology
Royal Prince Alfred Hospital
Sydney, Australia

HISTORY OF ARTERIAL DILATATION

Transluminal dilatation of stenotic lesions in atherosclerotic arteries was initially advocated by Dotter, in 1964. Dilatation was performed using successively larger coaxial polyethylene catheters (a 12F catheter over an 8F catheter). Staple and van Andel later used tapered-tip catheters of 5–12F diameter, to a similar effect. The taper configuration reduced trauma to the arterial wall, which had been a common problem with Dotter's blunt-nosed catheters.

Dotter postulated that a dilatation balloon technique would be required, and he successfully dilated a stenosed iliac artery using a Fogarty balloon embolectomy catheter in 1965. The concept of balloon dilatation was advanced greatly in 1974, when Gruntzig reported the use of a double-lumen polyvinyl balloon catheter.

Since that time, many advances have been made in the design and construction of angioplasty balloons. Stronger, non-compliant, non-elastomeric balloons have been developed, which can withstand high inflation pressures without distortion of shape or overstretching of diameter.

Early polyvinyl chloride balloons stretched easily with moderate pressure, whereas the more recent expandable polymer balloons are stronger and provide forceful radial dilatation of lesions. Increased catheter flexibility and decreased catheter diameters have improved the maneuvreability of devices; this means that they are able to cross tight regions of stenosis, including those in small tortuous arteries of the coronary circulation and the lower leg. The mechanisms of transluminal balloon angioplasty are depicted in Figs 4.1–4.3.

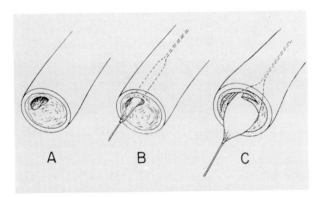

Fig. 4.1 Mechanism of balloon dilatation of an arterial stenosis. (a) Arterial stenosis. **(b)** The angioplasty balloon is positioned within the atherosclerotic narrowing. **(c)** The weakest point in the plaque is fractured by expansion of the balloon.

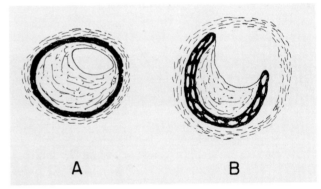

Fig. 4.2 Mechanism of dilatation of the arterial lumen by transluminal balloon angioplasty.

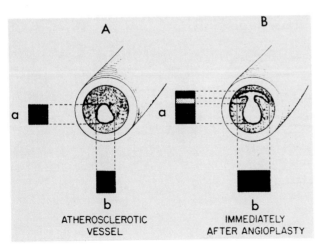

Fig. 4.3 Theoretical angiographic projections of an atherosclerotic vessel before and after successful angioplasty. Angiographically, the lumen appears enlarged in both projections **(a,b)**, but only in projection **(a)** can the split be seen. Projection **(a)** shows a segment that is less radiodense than projection **(b)**. (From Block, 1982, with permission.)

EQUIPMENT AND ANCILLARY INSTRUMENTS

The evolution of designs for balloon angioplasty and components of current catheters are shown in Figs 4.4–4.6.

Balloon catheters

The characteristics of a balloon catheter must be considered when choosing the appropriate equipment for a particular patient; these are as follows (Fig. 4.7):

1   Balloon diameter.

2   Balloon length.

3   Catheter diameter (usually 4–9F, but including new ultrathin catheters).

4   Catheter length (suitable for peripheral vascular or coronary access).

5   Catheter flexibility.

6   Profile and diameter of the catheter tip and deflated balloon (it should be capable of passing through the lumen of the stenotic region).

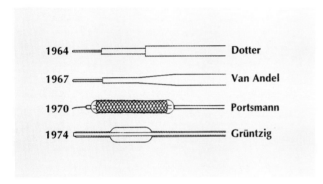

Fig. 4.4 Evolution of catheter design for percutaneous balloon angioplasty.

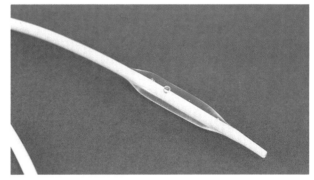

Fig. 4.5 Typical dual lumen design of an angioplasty balloon. The central lumen allows passage of a guidewire or injection of radiological contrast, while the outer lumen is used for inflation of the balloon, positioned close to the tip of the catheter.

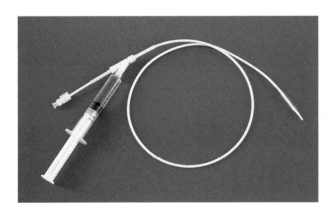

Fig. 4.6 Separate proximal ports for balloon inflation and guidewire. Decreased shaft size and deflated balloon profiles result in less entry site trauma and less resistance to the passage of the catheter through tight stenoses.

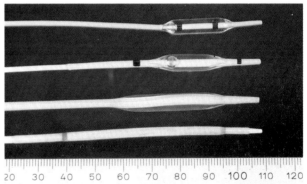

Fig. 4.7 Balloon catheters illustrating differences in catheter diameter, balloon diameter and balloon length.

Recent high pressure balloons may allow inflation to pressures of 12–15 atmospheres without an increase in diameter. This means that a greater dilating force is achieved without overexpansion; this characteristic may be particularly favourable in densely fibrotic, atherosclerotic stenoses.

A wide range of insertion needles, guidewires and diagnostic or interventional angiography catheters have been developed. Preshaped catheters and floppy-tipped wires give increased maneuvreability, and have expanded the range of vessels and lesions amenable to angioplasty (Fig. 4.8).

Guidewires

The ideal guidewire should be atraumatic – with a soft, shaped tip – steerable, and slippery (minimal friction). These features allow the guidewire to readily transmit torque, while being strong enough to cross the lesion so as to provide a sturdy track for the treatment balloon to follow. Wire strength and stiffness are closely related to diameter. There are six basic classifications of guidewire:

Standard guidewire

The basic construction is of a core wire inside an outer coiled spring. An outer bonded Teflon coating is usually applied to reduce friction. The standard guidewire is non-steerable and of varying stiffness, despite a distal taper which gives flexibility to the tip. However, it tends to be the most traumatic guidewire.

J-shaped guidewire

This may have a moveable inner core which can be retracted or extended, allowing the tip to bend and soften, or to extend.

Floppy-tip guidewire

This has no core wire in the distal 10–15 cm, conveying maximum flexibility.

Steerable guidewire

An angulated distal tip is combined with a stiff proximal shaft, to transmit torque and allow steerage of the leading end. A torque device may be fitted to the proximal shaft, facilitating rotation.

Exchange wire

A longer wire, 145–260 cm in length, allows the balloon catheter to be withdrawn and a new one loaded, without moving the distal portion of the wire from its safe position through the lesion.

Hydrophilic guidewire

Slippery guidewires, also known as 'eel' wires, are coated with a complex polymer which causes them to become very slick when wetted. This characteristic results in low friction between the guidewire and atherosclerotic lesions, as well as allowing easy passage of the balloon catheter over the wire.

In general, guidewires are used to find and secure a pathway through the artery and the stenotic

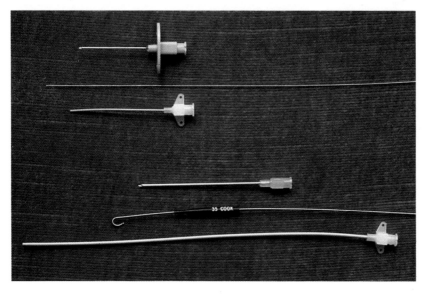

Fig. 4.8 Insertion needles, guidewires and diagnostic or interventional angiography catheters. A wide range of these instruments have been developed. Preshaped catheters and floppy-tipped wires give increased maneuvreability, and have increased the range of vessels and lesions amenable to angioplasty.

lesion. They pass well into the channel beyond and act as a guide to the subsequent passage of therapeutic devices.

Guiding catheters

Angiographic delivery or guiding catheters are used to provide support to the probing guidewire, when the lumen or route through a lesion is very tortuous. They are most valuable in conjunction with soft-tipped, torquable guidewires. They may also be used for localized injection of contrast

(Fig. 4.9).

A frequently used technique is to traverse a difficult lesion with a fine guidewire, load an angiography catheter over this wire to pass the lesion, and then change via the catheter to a more substantial guidewire that will support and direct the balloon catheter more effectively. A typical angiographic suite and procedure are shown in Figs 4.10 and 4.11; Figs 4.12–4.14 depict the actual mechanism of dilatation in an arterial specimen.

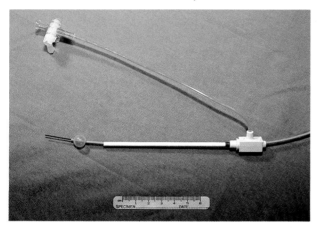

Fig. 4.9 Typical angioplasty sheath, with haemostatic proximal valve system and an injection sidearm. A balloon-tipped catheter has been fed through the lumen of the sheath.

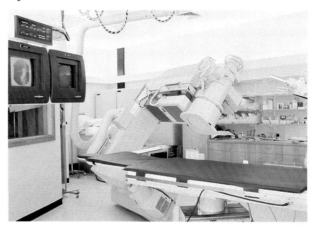

Fig. 4.10 Angiography suite suitable for angioplasty procedures. Rotating image intensifier allows viewing of different planes. The table allows screening of various segments of the arterial system.

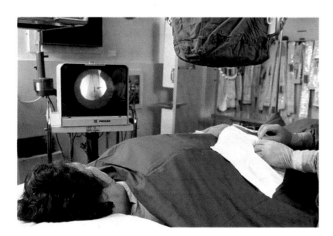

Fig. 4.11 Angioplasty procedure in progress. The patient is under local anaesthetic and mild sedation. Sterile technique is applied.

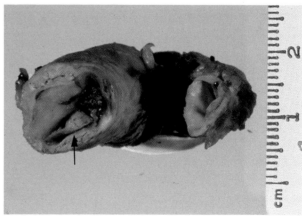

Fig. 4.12 Resected specimen of artery following unsuccessful angioplasty procedure. The process is essentially producing a controlled injury to the vessel wall, with dilatation of the lumen by cracking of atherosclerotic plaque and the layers of the wall. As is demonstrated here, early concepts of compressing the plaque were false – the plaque is still present but is disrupted by the cracks in its surface.

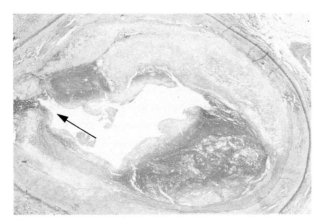

Fig. 4.13 Cross-sectional histology specimen of an artery after balloon angioplasty. The full thickness crack of the plaque and underlying vessel wall can be seen. LM, ×4.

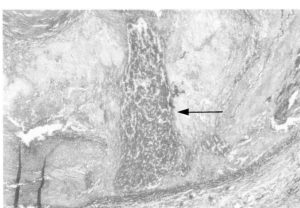

Fig. 4.14 Region of vessel wall trauma caused by dilatation, with recent thrombus in the cracked surface. The lesions that prove most resistant to angioplasty have densely elastic fibrosis or calcification that is very difficult to disrupt. LM, ×40.

ILIAC DILATATION

Fig. 4.15 Iliac dilatation: percutaneous transluminal angioplasty of the left iliac artery has been performed. The angiogram on the left shows several stenotic lesions of the common iliac and external iliac arteries. An excellent technical result is shown in the postdilatation film (right). Balloon angioplasty is especially effective for localized, short stenotic lesions (or short length occlusions) of the iliac arteries, with good rates of initial recanalization (> 90%) and long term patency. Cumulative patency rates of approximately 50–70% at the four-year interval have been reported. A retrograde femoral approach is usually employed, and frequently bilateral iliac angioplasty may be performed via one femoral access site. Less favourable lesions are those longer than 5 cm, total occlusions, or lesions associated with diffuse atherosclerotic disease and poor arterial runoff.

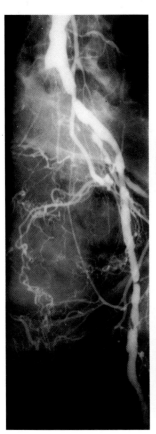
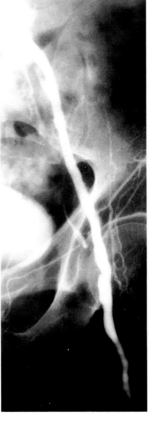

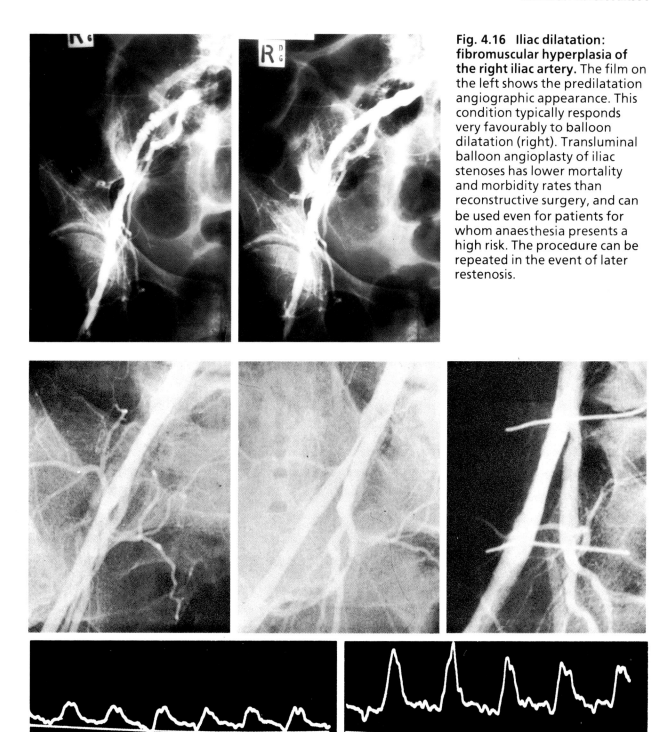

Fig. 4.16 Iliac dilatation: fibromuscular hyperplasia of the right iliac artery. The film on the left shows the predilatation angiographic appearance. This condition typically responds very favourably to balloon dilatation (right). Transluminal balloon angioplasty of iliac stenoses has lower mortality and morbidity rates than reconstructive surgery, and can be used even for patients for whom anaesthesia presents a high risk. The procedure can be repeated in the event of later restenosis.

Fig. 4.17 Iliac dilatation: measurement of pressure gradients. This may be very helpful in determining the success of an angioplasty procedure. In this case, the initial angiogram (left) of the left iliac segment appears satisfactory, but the measured pressure wave was abnormally dampened, with pressures significantly lower than the aortic pressure. An oblique view (centre) demonstrates the haemodynamically significant stenosis of the external iliac artery that had been concealed by overlap of the internal iliac artery. The widened lumen and improved pressures are seen in the postdilatation film (right). Pressure gradients across a lesion may be measured simultaneously with dual catheters, or separately by 'drawback' of a single catheter through the stenosis.

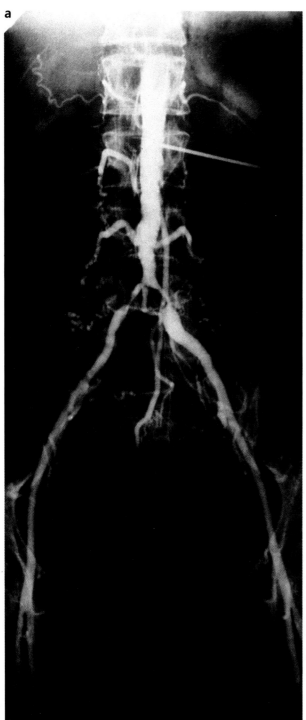

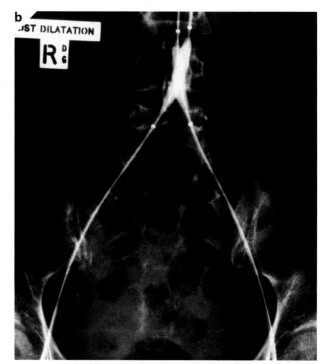

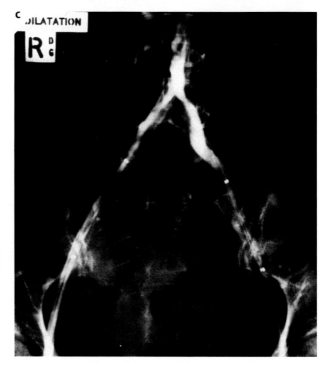

Fig. 4.18 Iliac dilatation: technique for percutaneous transluminal angioplasty of iliac lesions at the aortic bifurcation. (a) Tight stenotic lesions at the origin of both common iliac arteries. **(b)** Bilateral retrograde femoral catheterization has been performed, and the balloons are being inflated simultaneously to perform dilatation at the bifurcation area. This 'kissing balloon' technique helps prevent compression of the contralateral iliac artery orifice and reduces the incidence of resultant embolization. **(c)** Postdilatation appearance of the common iliac arteries. The external iliac segments show a degree of spasm resulting from the presence of the catheters. This is not uncommon, and it resolved spontaneously with return of excellent femoral pulses. Vasodilators may be administered intra-arterially, or systemically.

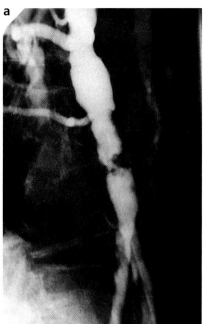
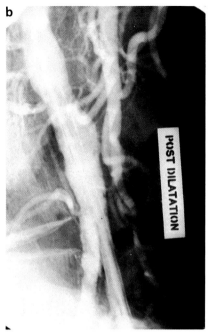

AORTIC DILATATION

Fig. 4.19 Aortic dilatation: transluminal dilatation of a stenotic lesion of the infrarenal abdominal aorta. (a) Aortogram in the lateral plane shows a tight stenosis which was poorly demonstrated on the anteroposterior film. **(b)** Excellent result after dilatation. The results in well selected aortic lesions are comparable to those achieved in the iliac segment, with good rates of initial recanalization and very successful long term patency.

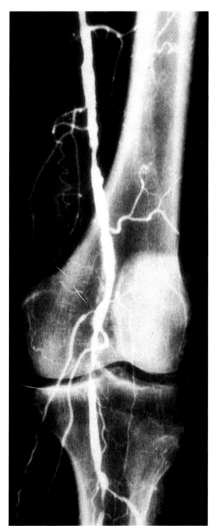
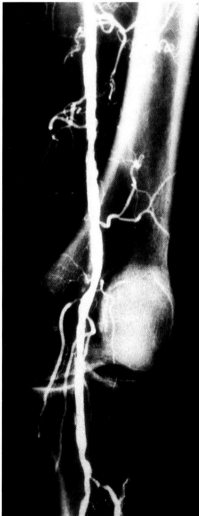

FEMORAL DILATATION

Fig. 4.20 Femoral dilatation: percutaneous transluminal angioplasty of several areas of the distal superficial artery and popliteal artery. Pre- (left) and post- (right) angiographic studies. The results of percutaneous angioplasty of infrainguinal arterial disease are not as good as for aortoiliac disease. In this site, if the angioplasty fails approximately 10% of patients are made clinically worse, usually with coincidental reduction of the ankle–brachial systolic blood pressure ratio. Favourable factors are for the lesion to be short, localized (as compared to generalized stenotic disease) and having good runoff below the knee. Stenotic lesions are more likely to be successfully treated, compared to total occlusions. Satisfactory results can be obtained if patients are carefully selected.

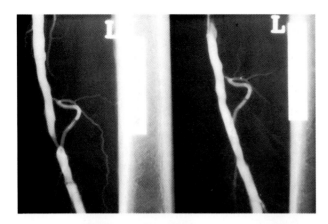

Fig. 4.21 Femoral dilatation: favourable lesion of the superficial femoral artery for successful transluminal dilatation. A localized, tight stenosis near the adductor canal level has a relatively unaffected proximal and distal vessel. The prospects of sustained long term patency are good.

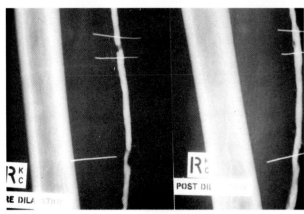

Fig. 4.22 Femoral dilatation: multiple lesions of superficial femoral artery. The disease process in this patient is more diffuse than that shown in Fig. 4.21, with consequent increased likelihood of early recurrent stenosis or occlusion. The atherosclerotic process may also progress to involve other segments of the vessel.

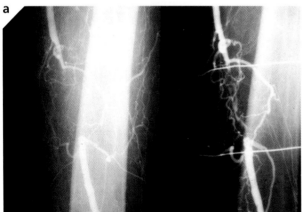

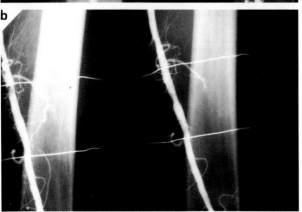

Fig. 4.23 Femoral dilatation: percutaneous transluminal angioplasty (PTA) of an occlusive lesion of the left superficial femoral artery. The lesion is 6 cm in length at the adductor canal level. **(a)** The proximal and distal extent of the occlusion are marked after injection of contrast. The radiopaque skin markers act as a guide for crossing of the lesion by a guidewire, and for subsequent positioning of the balloon for dilatation. **(b)** After initial dilatation, a satisfactory recanalization has been obtained, but a large residual plaque is seen near the proximal margin of the previously occluded segment (left). Repeat dilatation of this lesion gave a satisfactory result (right). The long term patency rates after PTA of femoral occlusions are inferior to patency after PTA of stenoses.

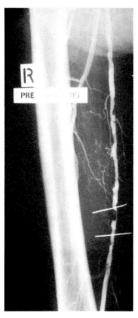 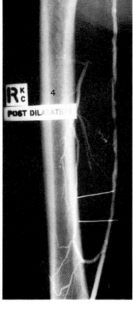 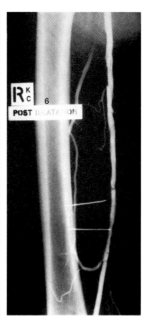

Fig. 4.24 Femoral dilatations: stenotic lesions of the right superficial femoral artery. Multiple lesions are seen, with radiopaque skin markers over the distal tightest stenotic lesion (left). After PTA with a 4 mm diameter balloon, the result is satisfactory but shows residual stenosis in several sites (centre). There is an improved result after dilatation with a larger, 6 mm diameter balloon (right).

POPLITEAL ANGIOPLASTY

SUBCLAVIAN ANGIOPLASTY

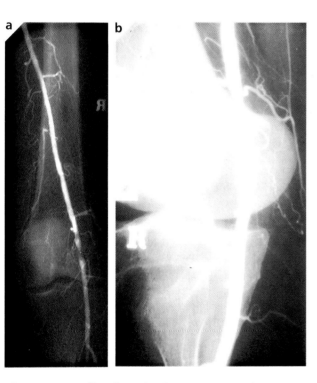

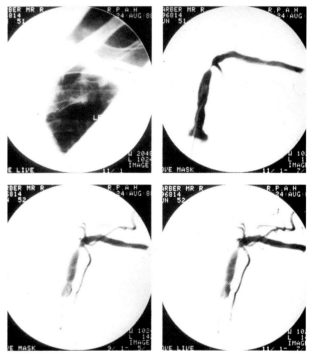

Fig. 4.25 Popliteal angioplasty: stenotic lesion of left popliteal artery. (a) Predilatation view just above level of knee joint. **(b)** Lateral post-dilatation view of treated vessel segment after successful angioplasty.

Fig. 4.26 Subclavian angioplasty: angiogram of subclavian artery in a patient with arm claudication associated with diminished brachial and radial pulses. Pre-angioplasty film (top right) shows tight stenosis of the left subclavian artery. Postdilatation views (below) demonstrate improved lumen with some residual stenosis. The vertebral artery was not demonstrated. The patient had an excellent clinical response.

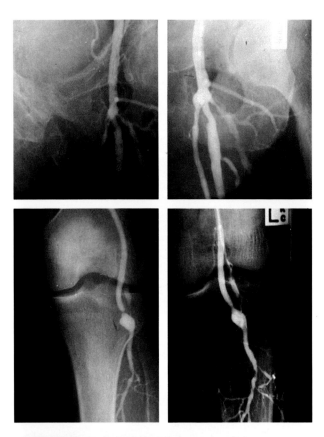

BALLOON ANGIOPLASTY OF SAPHENOUS VEIN BYPASS GRAFTS

Fig. 4.27 Balloon angioplasty of saphenous vein bypass grafts. This patient had recurrent claudication two years after placement of a femoral-distal popliteal saphenous vein bypass graft. Angiography (left, above and below) demonstrated two tight stenotic lesions of the graft near the proximal and distal anastomoses. Treatment with balloon angioplasty after direct puncture of the graft led to improvement of the stenotic lesions (right, above and below), with reappearance of the popliteal pulse and symptomatic improvement. Monitoring of saphenous vein graft haemodynamics by vascular laboratory duplex Doppler scanning is resulting in detection of stenotic lesions in these grafts, allowing treatment before occlusion occurs.

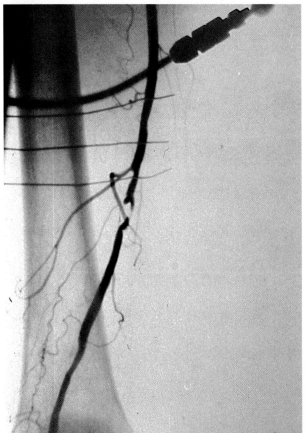

BALLOON ANGIOPLASTY COMBINED WITH ADJUNCTIVE FIBRINOLYTIC THERAPY

Fig. 4.28 Adjunctive use of intra-arterial fibrinolytic therapy (steptokinase or urokinase infusion) with subsequent angioplasty. This film shows the appearance of the superficial femoral artery after six hours of local fibrinolytic therapy which had been administered by arterial catheter. Thrombus overlying a stenotic plaque has been lysed, revealing the cause of the recent vascular occlusion, which was then successfully dilated. Fibrinolytic therapy may also be used for treatment of acute thrombosis which occurs as a complication of angioplasty attempts. In this situation, the recent non-organized thrombus is very susceptible to lysis by immediate local infusion of a fibrinolytic agent.

RENAL ARTERY DILATATION

Balloon dilatation can also be used to treat disease in the branches of the abdominal aorta, particularly the renal and mesenteric arteries. Renovascular disease is found to be the cause of hypertension in approximately 5% of hypertensive patients; it may often be amenable to dilatation, especially if there is a short, focal stenosis of the renal artery which does not involve the ostium.

Lesions of the orifice of the artery, formed by

an extension of aortic plaque, are less favourable and difficult to treat successfully, as are totally occlusive lesions of the renal artery (Figs 4.29–4.31).

With good patient selection, initial success rates of 90% can be expected for renal angioplasty, and long term studies have shown patency rates of 70–90% at one to five years. Recurrent renal artery stenosis is likely if an atherosclerotic lesion is dilated but shows a residual stenosis greater than 30% at the end of the procedure.

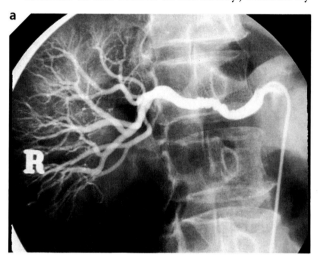

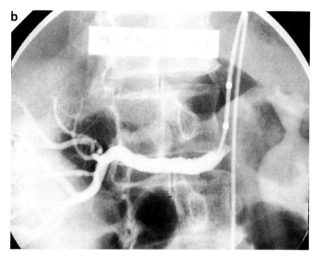

Fig. 4.29 (a) Pretreatment angiogram of the right kidney showing typical irregularity associated with fibromuscular hyperplasia. Access to the artery is usually obtained with a steerable, floppy-tip guidewire introduced through a retrograde femoral or axillary approach. Angulated guiding catheters may be helpful. Usually a short-length balloon on a 5F shaft is used. Localized infusion of heparin and vasodilators helps prevent spasm or occlusion. The lesions of fibromuscular hyperplasia

are often more tightly constricting than the angiogram suggests, but are very responsive to balloon angioplasty, and require less inflation pressure for adequate treatment than do the atherosclerotic lesions. (b) Postdilatation angiogram showing excellent result after angioplasty. Follow up studies have demonstrated that dilated lesions of the renal artery have a tendency to smooth out in time.

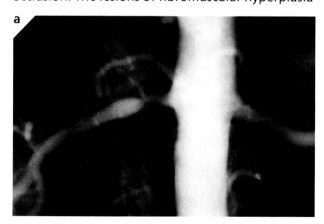

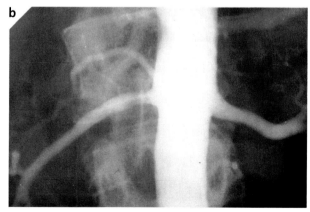

Fig. 4.30 Renal artery dilatation: stenotic lesion of right renal artery. (a) This lesion is suitable for

angioplasty. **(b)** Postdilatation film shows a satisfactory technical result.

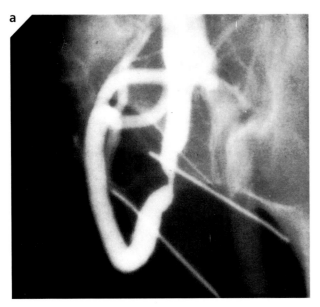

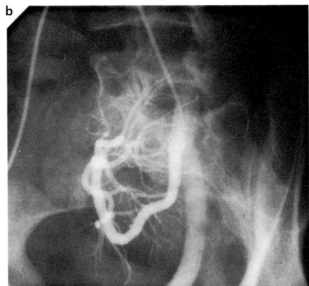

Fig. 4.31 Renal artery dilatation: transplanted kidney. Stenotic lesions of transplanted kidney arteries respond less well to angioplasty than do native renal arteries, and stenoses at the anastomosis are more difficult to treat than more distal lesions. Causes of transplant artery stenosis include an arterial kink associated with positioning the kidney in the iliac fossa, rejection

reactions, vessel trauma, extrinsic compression and haemodynamic disturbances. **(a)** Angiogram showing a stenotic area of the transplant renal artery which was associated with the development of hypertension. Successful dilatation was performed. **(b)** Postdilatation follow up study at an interval of two years shows good long term result.

BALLOON ANGIOPLASTY OF DIALYSIS FISTULA

Fig. 4.32 Balloon angioplasty of dialysis fistula. This shows successful percutaneous dilatation of a saphenous vein loop graft used for long term haemodialysis access in the forearm. Long term results of percutaneous transluminal angioplasty in dialysis fistulae are generally poor.

COMPLICATIONS OF BALLOON ANGIOPLASTY

The complications of percutaneous transluminal angioplasty are demonstrated in Figs 4.33–4.41, and are classified as follows (Table 4.1):

Complications of Balloon Angioplasty
At the arterial site Haemorrhage Haematoma, bruising False aneurysm Intimal flap, arterial occlusion Arteriovenous fistula Spasm **At the lesion** Failed procedure; inability to cross the lesion Failed procedure; inability to dilate Subintimal dissection or flap Arterial rupture, extravasation Thrombosis Residual stenosis Late or early recurrent stenosis **In the arterial segment proximal or distal to the lesion** Spasm Thrombosis Embolus Plaque or vessel wall trauma, dissection Arterial perforation

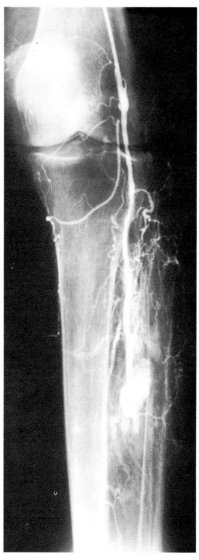

Fig. 4.34 Arterial perforation. Extravasation of contrast material is seen around the peroneal artery at the site of arterial perforation caused by guidewire manipulations. Perforation may also be caused by the guiding catheter or balloon, particularly with balloon overinflation and the resultant overdistension of the vessel. Severe bleeding is uncommon with perforation of vessels distal to the iliac level, and urgent operation is not usually required.

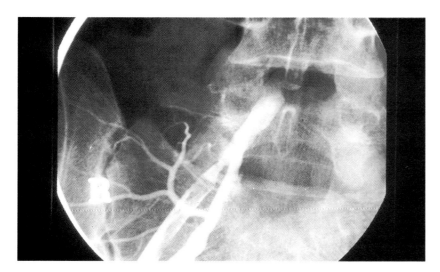

Fig. 4.33 Acute thrombosis. Thrombus is seen in the external iliac artery during angioplasty. Thrombotic complications are associated with vessel wall dissection or rupture, creation of an intimal flap, and difficult cannulation of tortuous or narrow vessels. Acute thrombosis can often be alleviated by infusion of thrombolytic medications via the angiography catheter directly into the clot, especially if the access site was via the contralateral femoral artery.

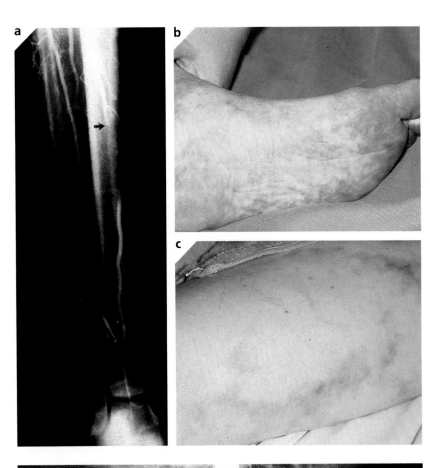

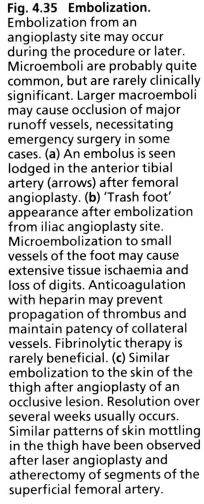

Fig. 4.35 Embolization.
Embolization from an angioplasty site may occur during the procedure or later. Microemboli are probably quite common, but are rarely clinically significant. Larger macroemboli may cause occlusion of major runoff vessels, necessitating emergency surgery in some cases. (a) An embolus is seen lodged in the anterior tibial artery (arrows) after femoral angioplasty. (b) 'Trash foot' appearance after embolization from iliac angioplasty site. Microembolization to small vessels of the foot may cause extensive tissue ischaemia and loss of digits. Anticoagulation with heparin may prevent propagation of thrombus and maintain patency of collateral vessels. Fibrinolytic therapy is rarely beneficial. (c) Similar embolization to the skin of the thigh after angioplasty of an occlusive lesion. Resolution over several weeks usually occurs. Similar patterns of skin mottling in the thigh have been observed after laser angioplasty and atherectomy of segments of the superficial femoral artery.

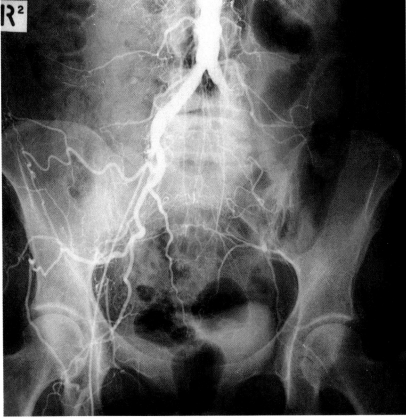

Fig. 4.36 Acute occlusion.
Percutaneous transluminal angioplasty of the left iliac artery was performed via retrograde approach from the right femoral. Acute occlusion resulted after balloon inflation, presumably due to dissection or creation of an intimal flap. Fibrinolytic therapy may be useful in this situation to clear the thrombus and reveal the nature of the lesion causing occlusion. Vascular stenting could prove a valuable adjunct in the salvage of complications such as this.

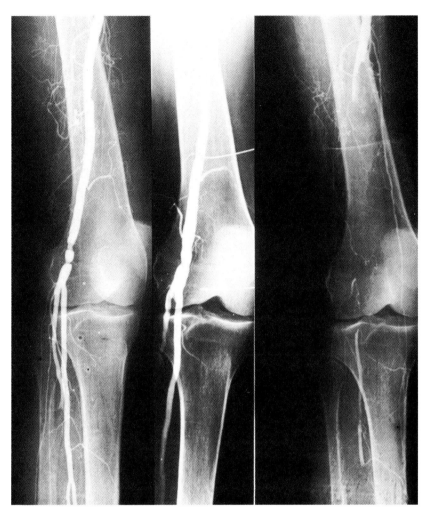

Fig. 4.37 Late failure. Series of angiograms demonstrating late failure after initial successful angioplasty of a stenotic lesion in the popliteal artery. The three films show the stenotic popliteal lesion (left), the immediate result after dilatation (middle), and the occluded segment of artery six months later (right). The last study was performed because of recurrent symptoms at this interval.

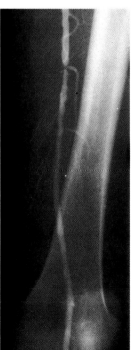
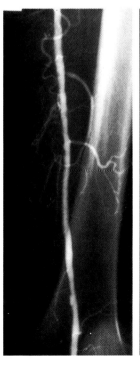
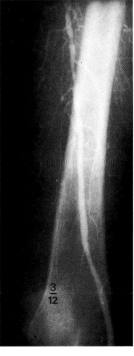

Fig. 4.38 Restenosis. Dilatation of a stenotic lesion of the superficial femoral artery (left) had a good initial result (middle), but recurrence of the lesion is seen at three months (right). The exact rates of restenosis or reocclusion of lesions after angioplasty are difficult to determine with confidence, because of variations in the given vessel, the status of runoff and persistence of risk factors, such as smoking, in the patient. Restenosis is usually due to fibrointimal hyperplasia, and is more common after dilatation of longer lesions, total occlusions and diffuse atherosclerotic disease. Restenosis is likely if a residual stenosis greater than 30% was left after the original PTA. There is little evidence that any presently known form of pharmacological or immunological treatment can prevent restenosis. Aspirin and dipyridamole may prevent thrombosis or embolization, and are widely used.

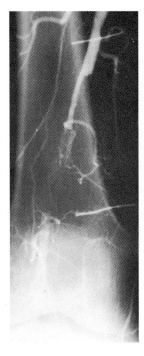
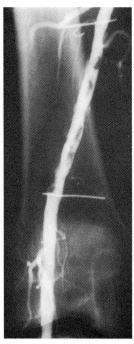
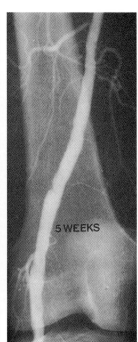

Fig. 4.39 Vessel wall dissection. An occlusion of the superficial femoral and popliteal arteries (left) was recanalized by percutaneous balloon angioplasty. The immediate angiogram monitoring shows extensive dissection planes into the plaque and arterial wall, with irregular opacification of the vessel lumen (middle). Healing and smoothing of the wall over five weeks is shown (right). The appearance of linear dissection planes in the wall, originally considered a complication of angioplasty, is now known to be a frequent accompaniment to successful dilatation, with the contrast in the wall being a consequence of efficient cracking of plaque.

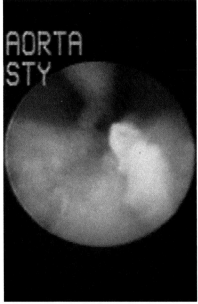
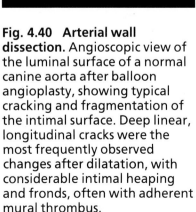

a

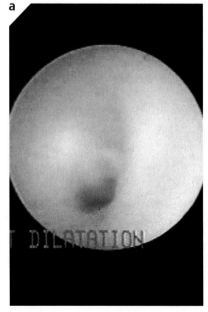

b

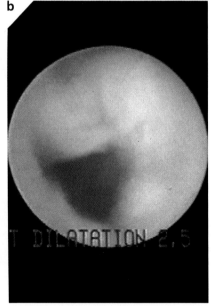

Fig. 4.40 Arterial wall dissection. Angioscopic view of the luminal surface of a normal canine aorta after balloon angioplasty, showing typical cracking and fragmentation of the intimal surface. Deep linear, longitudinal cracks were the most frequently observed changes after dilatation, with considerable intimal heaping and fronds, often with adherent mural thrombus.

Fig. 4.41 Angioscopic control of coronary artery dilatation. The lumen of the left anterior descending coronary artery (LAD) is shown in these endoscopic views obtained during the angioplasty procedure. **(a)** Angioscopic appearance of the LAD after balloon dilatation of a very tight stenosis with a 2 mm balloon.

The lumen has been improved but still shows significant residual stenosis. **(b)** After dilatation of the same region with a larger 2.5 mm balloon, considerable improvement in diameter was observed, with the lumen now considered adequate. Mild intimal trauma is seen after the angioplasty procedure.

EXTRUSION BALLOON DILATATION

New concepts in balloon delivery for transluminal dilatation have been developed. Modifications were made to help delivery of the balloon through lesions, and to decrease the incidence of complications due to dissection and perforation of highly stenotic or occlusive segments. The Fogarty–Chin extrusion balloon is an example of one of the newer concepts.

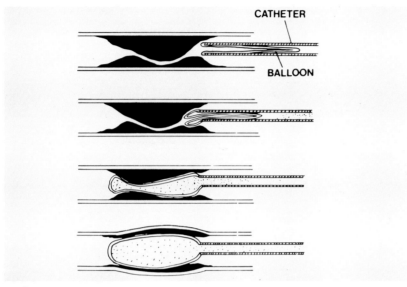

Fig. 4.42 Extrusion balloon dilatation. The Fogarty–Chin catheter. A polyethylene balloon initially inverted within the lumen of the catheter is unrolled throught the stenosis upon inflation. (From Chin and Fogarty, 1989, with permission.)

References

Block, P.C. *Progress in Cardiology, II.* Yu, P.N. and Goodwin, J.F. (1982) (eds) Lea & Febiger Philadelphia, PA, pp. 1–18.

Block, P.C., Mechanism of transluminal angioplasty (1984) *Am. J. Cardiol.,* **53**, 69C–71C.

Chin, A.K., Fogarty, T.J. (1989) Balloons and mechanical devices, In *Lasers in Cardiovascular Disease: Clinical Applications, Alternative Angioplasty Devices, and Guidance Systems* (eds R.A. White, W.S. Grundfest) Year Book Medical Publishers, Chicago, IL, pp. 217–27.

Dotter, C.T. (1980) Transluminal angioplasty: A long view. *Radiology,* **135**, 561–4.

Dotter, C.T., Judkins, M.P. (1964) Transluminal treatment of arteriosclerotic obstruction: Description of a new technic and a preliminary report of its application. *Circulation,* **30**, 654–70.

Fogarty, T.J., Chin, A., Shoor, P.S. *et al.* (1981) Adjunctive intraoperative arterial dilation: Simplified instrumentation technique. *Arch. Surg.,* **116**, 1391–8.

Gruntzig, A. (1978) Transluminal dilatation of coronary artery stenosis. *Lancet* (i) 263.

Gruntzig, A. and Hopff, H. (1974) Perkutane Rekanalisation chronischer arterieller Verschlusse mit einem neuen Dilatationskatheter: Modification der Dotter-Technik. *Dtsch. Med. Wochenschr.,* **99**, 2502–5.

Gruntzig, A., Senning, A., Siegenthaler, W.E. (1979) Nonoperative dilatation of coronary artery stenosis. N. Engl. J. Med. **30**, 61–8.

Katzen, B.T. (1984) Percutaneous transluminal angioplasty for arterial disease of the lower extremities. *AJR,* **142**, 23–5.

Ring, E.J., Freiman, D.B., McLean, G.K. and Schwartz, W. (1988) Percutaneous recanalization of common iliac artery occlusions: An unacceptable complication rate? *AJR,* **139**, 587–9.

Ring, E.J., McLean, G.K. and Freiman, D.B. (1982) Selected techniques in percutaneous transluminal angioplasty. *AJR,* **139**, 767–73.

Seldinger, S.I. (1953) Catheter placement of the needle in percutaneous arteriography. *Acta. Radiol.,* **39**, 368–76.

Staple, T.W. (1968) Modified catheter for percutaneous transluminal treatment of arteriosclerotic obstructions. *Radiology,* **91**, 1041–3.

Waltman, A.C., Greenfield, A.J., Novelline, R.A. *et al.* (1982) Transluminal angioplasty of the iliac and femoropopliteal arteries. *Arch. Surg.,* **117**, 1211–8.

Zimmerman, J.H. Fogarty, T.J. (1986) Adjunctive intraoperative dilatation (angioplasty), in *Vascular Surgery: Principles and Practice* (eds S.E. Wilson *et al.*) McGraw-Hill, Inc., New York, NY pp. 297–302.

5 Lasers

INTRODUCTION

The concept of using lasers to remodel stenotic lesions and recanalize arterial occlusions is based on the unique qualities of laser light.

The word 'laser' is an acronym for light amplification by stimulated emission of radiation, a concept initially described by Einstein in 1917. In the 1950s, this theory was reduced into practice with the development of the first industrial lasers. Currently, many of the early industrial prototypes, for example, carbon dioxide, argon and Nd:YAG, have been developed into commercially available units which are used in surgery. For this reason, these were the first lasers to be evaluated for cardiovascular tissue application. Many other prototypes are now becoming available, as special requirements to further develop this application are identified.

LASER BIOPHYSICS

Laser energy can be defined by particle (photons or quantums of energy) or wave theories. According to the wave theory, laser energy encompasses a wavelength range of 100 nm to approximately 1 mm on the electromagnetic spectrum (Fig. 5.1).

Laser energy has three unique characteristics: it is monochromatic, directional and coherent. Monochromicity means that the laser energy consists of a defined wavelength. If the wavelength is

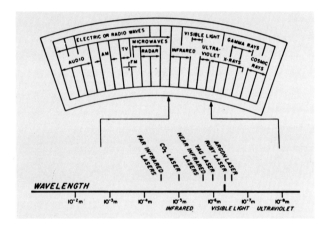

Fig. 5.1 Electromagnetic spectrum highlighting the wavelengths of laser energy. Laser energy is emitted from the ultraviolet (100–380 nm), through the visible (380–700 nm), to the infrared (700 nm–1 mm) wavelengths. (From White, 1988, with permission; modified with permission from Absten, 1988.)

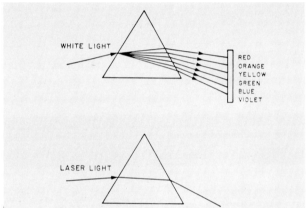

Fig. 5.2 Monochromicity of laser energy. White light passed through a prism produces a rainbow pattern as the individual wavelengths are separated. Laser light has only one wavelength, thus only one colour is produced. (From White, 1988, with permission.)

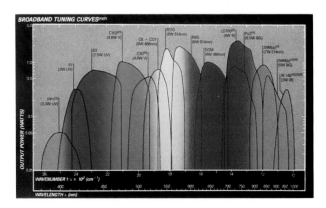

Fig. 5.3 Wavelength and power output for various dyes in a pumped dye laser. Each peaked curve represents the range produced by individual dyes.

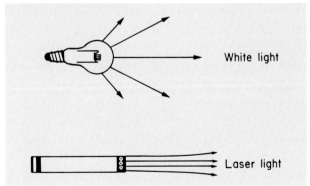

Fig. 5.4 Directionality of laser energy. (From White, 1988, with permission.)

in the visible range, then the energy is called 'light' and produces an intense colour corresponding to the particular wavelength. Normal white light from a source such as a lamp contains the entire spectrum of wavelengths of visible light. When white light is directed through a prism, the individual wavelengths are separated, producing the corresponding colours in a rainbow pattern. When laser light is passed through a prism, only one wavelength of the rainbow (i.e. one colour) is visible (Fig. 5.2).

Ideally, a laser should be tunable over the entire spectrum of wavelengths, with a range of available powers. At present, this capacity does not exist. Dye lasers use various organic dyes as lasing media, to produce a tunable characteristic over a range of approximately 300–1000 nm, but currently they are far from the idealized laser described above. Each dye produces wavelengths over a spectrum of approximately 100 nm or less.

The dyes can be cumbersome to handle, and some are unstable (Fig. 5.3).

The free electron laser is theoretically tunable over all wavelengths of the electromagnetic spectrum, but at present this requires a very large and expensive particle separator. Table 5.1 lists some of the available medical lasers that are being used both experimentally and clinically for surgical applications.

Laser light is also described as directional (Fig. 5.4). Directionality, or collimation, means that the laser energy is released in a highly concentrated, parallel beam, with minimal amounts of light spread. For example, light emitted from a light bulb is not directional, and spreads so as to light up the whole room. In contrast, laser light emitted in a dark room illuminates only a very small spot, the same size as that of the laser light source.

Table 5.1 Lasers used for medical applications		
Type of laser	**Wavelength (nm)**	
CO_2	10 000	
Hydrogen fluoride	2950	
Er:YAG	2940	
Nd:YAG	1320	Infrared
	1064	
Gallium arsenide	904	
Ruby	694 (red)	
Helium neon	632 (red)	
Tunable dye	628 (red)	
	577 (yellow)	
Gold	628 (red)	
Copper	578 (yellow)	Visible
	511 (green)	
Frequency-doubled Nd:YAG	532 (green)	
Argon	515 (green)	
	488 (blue)	
Excimer		
XeF	351	
KrF	248	
		Ultraviolet
ArF	193	

From White (1988) with permission.

The third unique property of laser energy is its coherence. According to the wave theory of electromagnetic radiation, the waveform of laser energy can be characterized according to wavelength, amplitude and frequency (Fig. 5.5). Amplitude is the ventricle height of the wave, wavelength (λ) is the distance between two successive wave peaks, and frequency (f) is the inverse of the wavelength with the velocity (v) of light being 186 000 miles per second ($v = \lambda f$).

The light waves emitted from a normal lamp are incoherent in that the waveforms have different amplitudes, different frequencies, and are not spatially aligned with identical peaks and valleys. Laser energy is coherent in that all of the waveform amplitudes, frequency and temporal distribution of the peaks and valleys of the curves are the same (Fig. 5.6).

The most important parameter to describe the overall laser-tissue interaction and enable quantitation of the amount of energy distributed so that a particular interaction is reproducible, is the power density or energy fluence. These two terms are used interchangeably in the literature, and may be referred to as 'fluence'. The energy fluence is described in Joules per square centimetre (J/cm^2), and the equation is as follows:

$$\text{Energy fluence } (J/cm^2) = \frac{\text{laser power output (W)} \times \text{exposure time (s)}}{\text{laser beam cross sectional area } (cm^2)}$$

LASER DELIVERY SYSTEMS

There are several characteristics of laser delivery systems that have an important effect on the energy delivered to the tissue interface. These include the method of energy delivery (fibreoptic, articulating arm, waveguide, etc.), focus of the laser energy and mode of delivery (continuous wave, pulsed, etc.).

To enable precise delivery of laser energy at some distance from the source, such as the operating table, flexible delivery systems are desirable. For certain types of lasers (Nd:YAG, argon, dye)

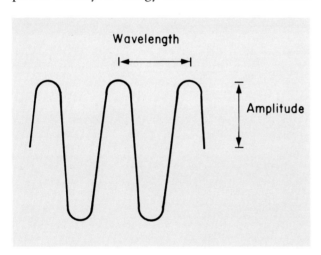

Fig. 5.5 Wave theory of laser energy. (From White, 1988, with permission.)

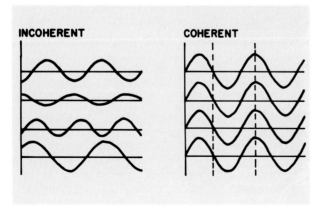

Fig. 5.6 Incoherent versus coherent waveforms. (From White, 1988, with permission.)

this is easily accomplished with quartz fibreoptics (Fig. 5.7).

For wavelengths that are absorbed by the quartz fibre or destroyed by high-peak energies, such as carbon dioxide laser energy, current delivery is by articulating arms or hollow waveguides (Fig. 5.8).

In most cases, the fibreoptic delivery systems absorb approximately 10–20% of the laser energy. The amount of energy transmitted also varies with the wavelength of the light, fibre diameter and shape of the fibre tip. Upon transmission through the fibre, the collimated laser light changes in direction so that divergence of the laser light at the tip of the fibre is approximately 10–15° in most fibres (Fig. 5.9). An advantage of the articulated arm delivery for carbon dioxide is that the collimation of energy is unaffected, although the arms are somewhat cumbersome to use and are not suitable for endoscopic delivery.

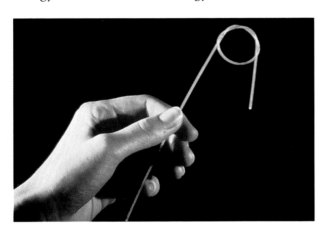

Fig. 5.7 Optic fibre, used to transmit laser energy to the target site.

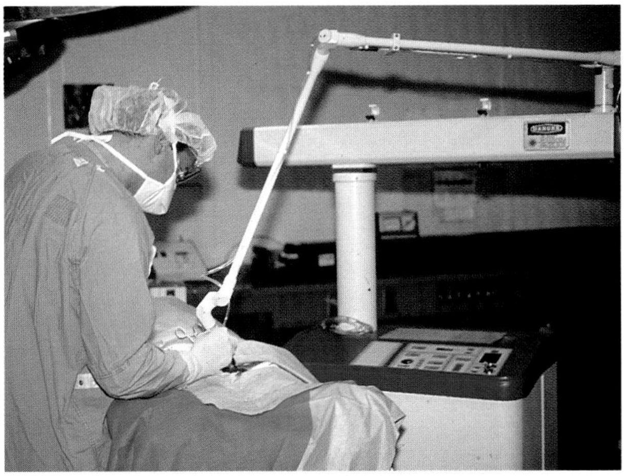

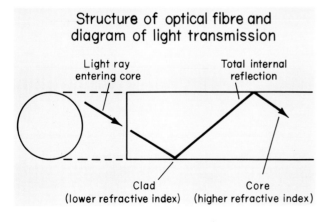

Fig. 5.8 Articulating arm, used to deliver carbon dioxide laser energy.

Fig. 5.9 Transmission of laser energy by an optic fibre. Schematic representation.

Structure of optical fibre and diagram of light transmission

Light ray entering core

Total internal reflection

Clad (lower refractive index)

Core (higher refractive index)

LASER SAFETY

Establishing and maintaining a laser safety programme is mandatory in each laser-operating facility. Such a programme should include methods of obtaining approvals for credentials, use of devices, definition of facility specifications, in-service training and continuing education. Lasers can cause eye damage, skin burns and combustion of flammable materials, as well as being a significant risk in electrical accidents since many of these instruments require high power supplies.

In order to assure the safety of personnel and patients, laser rooms must have all windows covered with non-transparent barriers to prevent inadvertent passage of laser light. All doors should provide restricted access to the room during laser activation, with clearly visible warning signs and flashing lights to signify that the system is activated (Figs 5.10–5.12).

Laser energy can affect different parts of the eye, depending on the structure absorbing a particular wavelength. The three most vulnerable areas are the cornea, lens and retina. Laser energy outside the visible range (<350 nm and >1400 nm) is absorbed by the cornea and lens; exposure can produce cataracts and corneal scarring. Laser energy in the visible wavelength is focused by the cornea and lens onto the retina, leading to up to a 100 000-fold amplification of radiation exposure.

Misdirection of the laser light even at low power can result in instantaneous burning of the retina and consequent blindness in the visual field corresponding to the burn spot. Everyone in the operating room, including the patient, must have

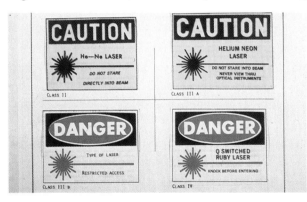

Fig. 5.10 Examples of laser warning signs for various classes of lasers.

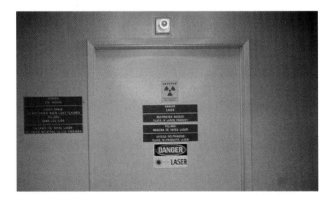

Fig. 5.11 Door to a laser facility. This should be clearly marked with warning signs and flashing lights which are activated when the system is in use.

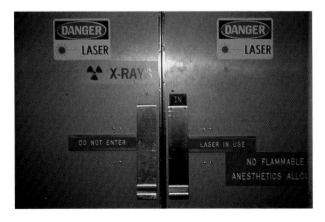

Fig. 5.12 Operating room doors adapted for laser use.

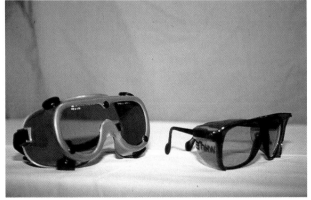

Fig. 5.13 Protective eyewear for laser procedures. Goggles or glasses with side shields are required, with lenses that are non-transparent to the wavelengths of different types of laser.

appropriate eyewear for each laser procedure (Fig. 5.13).

LASER-TISSUE INTERACTIONS

When laser energy interacts with the tissue surface, it may be absorbed, transmitted, scattered or reflected (Fig. 5.14). When laser energy interacts with tissue, the effects are dependent upon the way the energy is dissipated and the absorption characteristics of tissue for a particular wavelength of energy.

Laser energy can be described according to the wave theory, that is, as having a wavelength and a frequency. Laser energy may also be described as particles or photons with each having a quantum of energy corresponding to a particular wavelength. Garrison and Srinivasan have proposed a theory to explain the different tissue effects of absorbed laser energy. If the photons of laser light do not have enough energy to break chemical bonds, they cause vibration and collision of nearby atoms producing heat – a photothermal effect. This results in tissue burning and vapourization if enough energy is delivered. If the emitted photons have enough energy to break chemical

bonds, tissue ablation occurs by ionization of atoms and molecules – a photoablative or photochemical effect. The quantum of energy absorbed by the atom may also be re-emitted as photons with the same or less energy than those that were absorbed – laser-induced fluorescence (Fig. 5.15).

At present, this theory of photon energy absorption is used to explain the different laser-tissue interactions seen with different wavelengths of energy (Fig. 5.16). A single photon of ultraviolet light has sufficient energy to break one chemical bond, causing expansion and ejection of molecules without significant generation of heat.

Currently available instruments in most operating rooms are carbon dioxide, argon and Nd:YAG lasers. These are being used to cut, coagulate, ablate or fuse tissues, depending on the type of laser, mechanism of tissue interaction and amount of energy delivered. The carbon dioxide laser is primarily absorbed by water at the tissue surface. For this reason, it is useful for cutting applications because it rapidly vapourizes the water and tissue at the surface. The argon laser energy penetrates more deeply than carbon dioxide (440–800 μm), and it is absorbed primarily by chromagens such as haemoglobin or melanin.

Fig. 5.14 Laser-tissue interactions. (From White, 1988, with permission.)

Fig. 5.15 Possible mechanisms of laser-tissue interactions. (From White, 1988, with permission.)

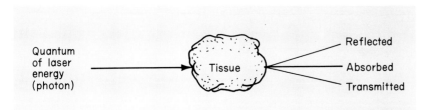

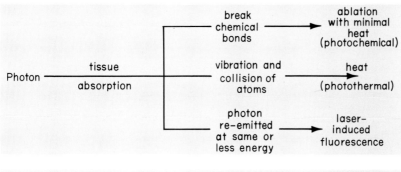

Fig. 5.16 Wavelength-specific effects of lasers on tissue. (From White, 1988, with permission.)

As with the continuous wave carbon dioxide lasers, the argon mechanism is primarily through heating and vapourization of tissue elements. Because of its selective absorption, the argon laser has been widely used for coagulation of pigmented and haematomatous lesions.

The Nd:YAG laser is not particularly well absorbed by any tissue elements, thus it penetrates deeply (1–4 mm) and is used primarily for tissue coagulation and necrosis (Fig. 5.17).

The mode of energy delivery (continuous wave or pulsed) has a significant effect on tissues. Continuous wave lasers deliver a constant power over intervals of a few tenths of a second to several seconds. Pulsed lasers deliver energy over a much shorter interval measured in nanoseconds (10^{-9} sec) or microseconds (10^{-6} sec), while the intensity of a pulsed laser is much higher than typically achievable from a continuous wave device. The energy per pulse is small, measured in millijoules (mJ), but the peak powers are high (megawatts)

leading to rapid ablation at the tissue interface. The repetition rate of pulses of energy is measured in Herz (Hz).

Both continuous wave and pulsed lasers can be mechanically 'chopped' or 'Q-switched' into a pulsed mode, by stopping the energy through a shutter mechanism, then releasing it over a very short interval (Fig. 5.18). In the Q-switch mode, the energy builds up very rapidly and can be released in a very short interval, with an intensity increased by several orders of magnitude. For several applications of laser energy, such as intraluminal ablation of atherosclerotic obstructions, it may be desirable to have tissue ablation without concomitant thermal injury to adjacent tissues. As described, most continuous wave lasers operate by having the energy absorbed and dissipated primarily as heat. Current research with new phototype lasers suggests that certain pulsed forms of energy may be capable of ablating tissue without producing significant thermal injury. In

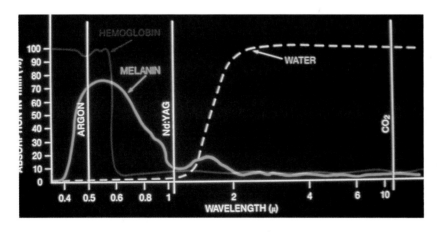

Fig. 5.17 Differential tissue component absorption by argon, Nd:YAG and carbon dioxide lasers. These features are responsible for the selected application of these lasers in surgical procedures.

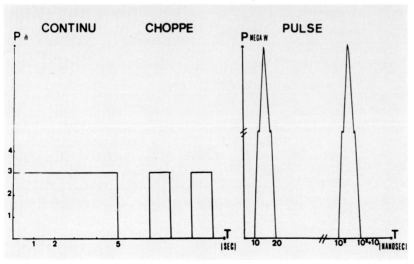

Fig. 5.18 Mode of energy delivery of continuous wave and pulsed lasers. Continuous wave lasers deliver constant power, usually in the range of several watts during a few seconds. The beam can be 'chopped' into constant power pulses. Pulsed-mode lasers deliver triangular-shaped pulses with a peak power in the range of megawatts, with the duration of approximately 10^{-9} The repetition rate of lasers is usually below 100 Hz; in this particular case this is 10 Hz. (From Steg and Menasche, 1989, with permission.)

some cases, it is thought that a photochemical breakdown of tissue occurs because high energy is absorbed by specific chemical bonds.

Photochemical ablation can be very precise. Of particular interest with regard to photochemical tissue ablation are the pulsed ultraviolet (excimer or ultraviolet YAG lasers) (Fig. 5.19).

It has been well documented that pulsed energy

from certain types of lasers at a low repetition rate can assimilate the postulated photochemical effect of ultraviolet systems. Thermal injury can be avoided even with certain types of lasers which ablate by a thermal mechanism, if the time of thermal diffusion of the tissue is less than the pulse interval (Fig. 5.20). Absence of thermal injury is accomplished only at relatively high peak

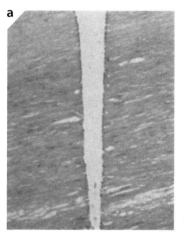 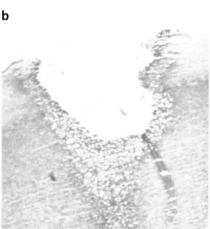 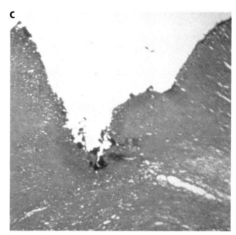

Fig. 5.19 Comparison of histological effects of three different lasers on atherosclerotic aorta. (a) A cut in human atherosclerotic aorta is made using a 308 nm excimer laser from a fibreoptic waveguide with 300 mJ/mm² and 40 nsec pulses. The thickness of this particular aorta is approximately 2.2 mm. The width at the very top is 0.4 mm, and the average width is approximately 0.35 mm. The crater walls are sharp, without carbonization or blast damage. A 2 μm rim of eosinophilic tissue is present, but adjacent tissue is not affected. **(b)** Effects of the Nd:YAG laser ablating atherosclerotic tissue which is only minimally calcified. The fibreoptic waveguide is

aimed perpendicularly to the intimal aortic surface, with 30 W for 25 sec over a 0.6 mm area. The crater is 2.1 mm in diameter by approximately 1.8 mm in depth. Note the surrounding zone of vacuolized tissue, carbonized edges and loss of tissue architecture. **(c)** Histological section of atherosclerotic aorta from a human cadaver, after irradiation with an argon laser using a 0.4 mm fibreoptic waveguide with the energy set at 5 W, spot size 0.5 mm for 2 sec. The crater created was 2.2 mm in diameter by approximately 1.6 mm in depth. Note the carbonization and lateral coagulation injury. (From Grundfest et al., 1987, with permission.)

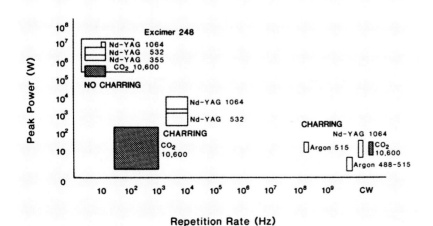

Fig. 5.20 Relationship between energy profile and tissue injury. Absence of thermal injury ('no scarring') is accomplished only at relatively high peak power and relatively low repetition rate. (From Isner, 1989, with permission.)

power and relatively low repetition rate; Figs 5.21 and 5.22 demonstrate this finding in myocardium. The effect of pulse characteristics on tissue ablation with the holmium:YAG (2150 nm) laser is demonstrated in Fig. 5.23.

In order to provide reproducible laser-tissue interactions via fibreoptic delivery, the depth of tissue penetration for any particular wavelength is required in addition to the parameters which have been discussed. Fig. 5.24 demonstrates that the ultraviolet wavelengths (up to 380 nm) provide precise tissue ablation due to the photochemical tissue ablation and shallow depth of penetration (2–4 mm). From 380 nm to approximately 2000 nm tissue penetration is much deeper, i.e. up to 2–4 nm for the ND:YAG laser at 1060 nm. Above 2000 nm penetration is again very shallow,

permitting a precise ultraviolet-like ablation.

Methods of enhancing laser delivery

In order to capture the laser energy at specific target sites, there are three main areas which are being developed to enhance laser delivery. Target specificity is being improved using radiological, ultrasound and spectroscopic techniques, described in more detail in subsequent chapters. The radiological method is used for most clinical studies. Angioscopic delivery is used to perform tissue ablation under direct vision, with the laser fibre being passed through a separate channel in an angioscope.

Intravascular ultrasound appears to be the most promising method; it allows precise guidance of devices through the vessel lumen by pro-

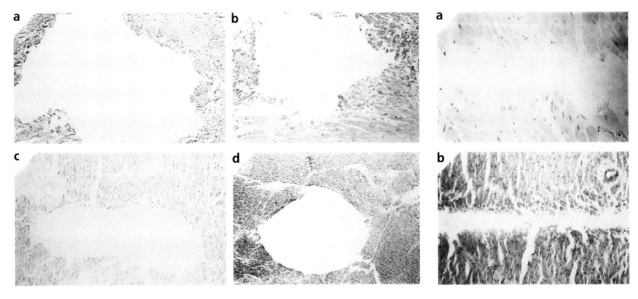

Fig. 5.21 Light microscopic findings following pulsed laser irradiation with low repetition rate. Neither of the typical light microscopic signs of thermal injury are observed after pulsed laser irradiation with: **(a)** Nd:YAG (532 nm, 10 Hz, 3 sec exposure, 350 mJ); **(b)** Nd:YAG (1064 nm, 10 Hz, 7 sec exposure, 190 mJ); **(c)** excimer (248 nm, 10 Hz, 5 sec exposure, 250 mJ); **(d)** carbon dioxide 'TEA' (10 600 nm, 180 mJ, 10 Hz, pulse duration: 1 μsec). H&E: **(a)** ×25; **(b)** ×25; **(c)** ×4; **(d)** ×29. (From Isner, 1989, with permission.)

Fig. 5.22 Light microscopic findings following pulsed laser ablation of myocardium. This was submerged in 5 mm of blood. **(a)** Section of specimen irradiated with pulsed ultraviolet light delivered as focused beam. There are no signs of thermal injury on either side of the laser ablation trough. H&E: ×101. **(b)** Light microscopic findings following carbon dioxide ('TEA') laser ablation of myocardium. The perimeter of laser ablation trough is free of thermal injury. H&E: ×64. (From Isner, 1989, with permission.)

viding visualization of both the luminal and transmural anatomy of the wall.

Spectroscopic analysis relies on the principle that tissues not only absorb laser energy but also re-emit the energy at a different wavelength. Preliminary evidence suggests that the pattern of re-emitted energy from a particular laser may be tissue-specific. Normal blood vessels have spectroscopic patterns that are different from atherosclerotic blood vessels. Thus, spectroscopic analysis may be useful in enhancing the target specificity of laser energy (Fig. 5.25).

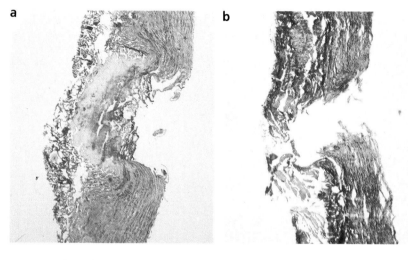

Fig. 5.23 Modification of the degree of residual thermal damage using a holmium:YAG laser at different energy parameters delivered to the intimal surface of fresh canine femoral artery. (a) Marked thermal effect with 6 Hz, 100 250 μsec pulses, 184 mJ/mm^2. **(b)** Minimal thermal effect noted by coagulation in the adventitia, otherwise relatively clean tissue ablation with 6 Hz, 50,100 nsec pulses of Q-switched energy at 300 mJ/mm^2.

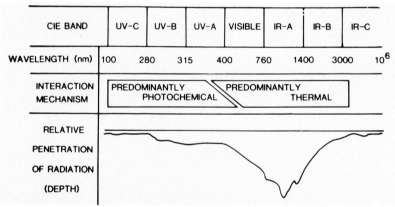

Fig. 5.24 Interaction mechanisms. Tissue interaction mechanisms are predominantly thermal for long wavelengths, and photochemical for shorter wavelengths. Attenuation is the combined effect of scattering and absorption, and defines the depth of penetration. (From Sliney, 1985, with permission.)

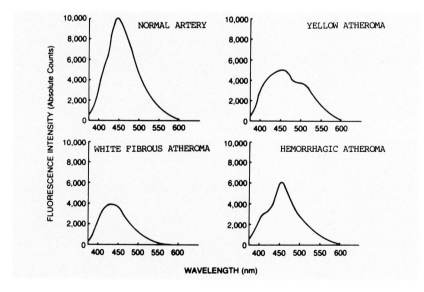

Fig. 5.25 Fluorescence spectra of human aorta excited with helium-cadmium laser (325 nm). Different patterns obtained in normal vessels and different types of atheroma are shown. (From Leon et al., 1988, with permission.)

Chromophores are also used to enhance local tissue absorption, resulting in a more specific tissue ablation. A chromophore is a substance that specifically absorbs a particular laser wavelength. Carotenoids (endogenous fats) are chromophores present in early atherosclerotic lesions, selectively absorbing the 460–480 nm wavelength. Tetracycline absorbs the 355 nm wavelength, and haematoporphyrin derivative (HPD) or its concentrated form, photofrin II, selectively absorbs argon laser energy.

HPD has several unique characteristics and demonstrates the potential application of chromophores. This compound has an affinity for vascular structures, binding to mitochondria and plasma membrane of the cell. Upon absorbing the argon light, HPD fluoresces pink and causes cell death by singlet oxygen toxicity. HPD is absorbed by atheroma and certain types of tumours, and is currently being evaluated for selective ablation of these tissues (Fig. 5.26).

EVOLUTION OF LASER ANGIOPLASTY

Laser angioplasty is a rapidly evolving technology. Since the first clinical trials in 1984, many different systems have been developed. Although

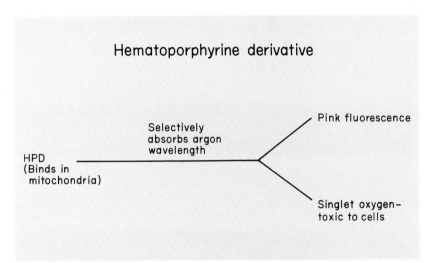

Fig. 5.26 Mechanism of action of haematoporphyrin derivative.

Table 5.2 Endovascular surgery modalities			
	Mechanism	**Applicable to**	**Advantages**
Thrombolysis	Clot lysis	Thromboses of variable lengths	Thrombosis removal without a surgical procedure
Balloons	Lesion displacement	Stenoses and short occlusions	Cost-effective percutaneous angioplasty
Lasers	Tissue ablation	Stenoses and occlusions	Tissue removal Miniature delivery systems
Atherectomy	Tissue removal	Stenoses and some occlusions	Tissue removal

this new technology has had less than a decade of development, promising preliminary data are being reported. As might be expected, significant limitations are also being identified to be addressed in future prototype devices.

Lasers are appealing for angioplasty in that precise tissue ablation can be accomplished via small fibreoptic delivery systems (200–600 µm diameter). The potential for laser angioplasty compared to other cardiovascular surgical techniques in treating atherosclerotic lesions is demonstrated in Table 5.2.

The initial trials of laser angioplasty, using free emission of argon or Nd:YAG continuous-wave energy via fibreoptics, demonstrated the ability to ablate atherosclerotic lesions, but the technique was limited by a significant rate of vessel perforation from excessive thermal damage. As a solution to this problem, an ovoid metal cap was attached to the end of the fibreoptic to limit the diffusion of heat and eliminate some of the perforations caused by the sharp fibre tip (Fig. 5.27).

The metal 'hot-tip' heats rapidly to approximately 1000°C in air when energized by the laser (Fig. 5.28).

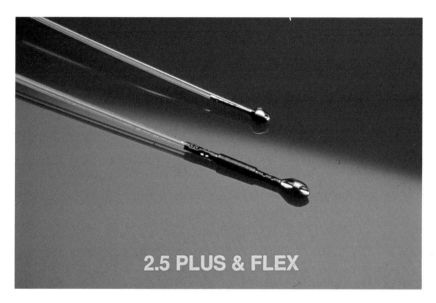

Fig. 5.27 Laser angioplasty. Ovoid metal cap, attached to the end of the optic fibre to limit the diffusion of heat and eliminate some of the perforations caused by the sharp fibre tip.

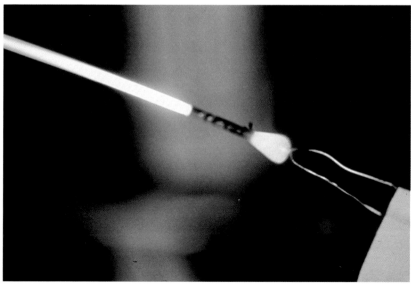

Fig. 5.28 Laser angioplasty. The metal 'hot tip' heats rapidly to approximately 1000°C when energized by the laser in air.

The temperatures achieved within the vessel lumen during angioplasty procedures have been reported to range from approximately 150°C to 400°C. Recent studies suggest that softer, fibrous lesions recanalize at temperatures of approximately 150°C, while calcified areas require temperatures of 250°C or greater. These data are currently being evaluated as a means to determine the variable resistance of lesions and possibly improve recanalizations by identifying sites that may require more extensive therapy. In addition, preintervention ultrasound characterization of lesions, i.e. fibrous or calcified, may be useful in determining which lesions are appropriate for laser-thermal therapy.

The initial clinical evaluations of the laser-thermal angioplasty systems were performed using 1.5 and 2.0 mm diameter hot-tips on a 600 μm fibreoptic. The studies were designed to compare the efficiency and safety of the technique with the conventional, approved balloon angioplasty methods. Approximately 60% of the procedures were performed on stenotic femoropopliteal lesions (this was chosen as a low-risk site for preliminary studies), and no attempt was made to compare the technique to standard surgical procedures, i.e. femoropopliteal bypass. Since the laser probes create a channel smaller than the size of the metal cap (channel size is estimated to be 60–70% of the tip diameter), recanalizations were followed by balloon dilatation to further enlarge the lumen. Thus, the technique is correctly termed laser-thermal-assisted balloon angioplasty (Fig. 5.29).

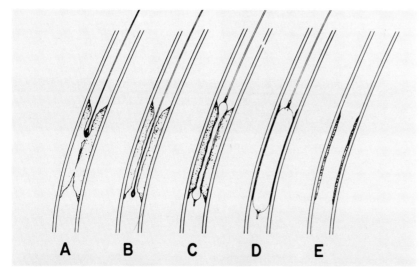

Fig. 5.29 Laser thermal-assisted balloon angioplasty. A, B: Recanalization of arterial occlusion by passage of the activated 'hot tip'. **C, D**: Balloon dilatation of the recanalized segment. **E**: Idealized result. (From White and White, 1989a, with permission.)

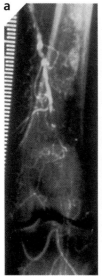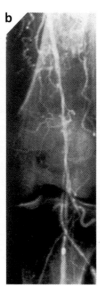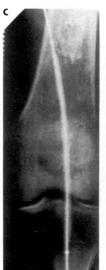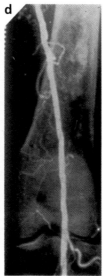

Fig. 5.30 Laser probe angioplasty in a 74-year-old woman with intermittent claudication. (a) A 9 mm occlusion of the left popliteal artery, not traversable with guidewire; ankle/arm systolic ratio: 0.35. **(b)** The probe has traversed the lesion (arrow), producing a moderate luminal channel. **(c)** Balloon dilating the involved segment. **(d)** A definitive lumen is produced by balloon dilatation; ankle/arm systolic pressure ratio: 0.72. Good clinical results were maintained at eight months follow up. (From Cumberland et al., with permission.)

Impressive preliminary reports of successful recanalizations using the laser-thermal devices, such as the case depicted in Fig. 5.30, lead to optimism regarding the utility of this method.

Following the initial multicentre experience in 219 peripheral arteries in ten institutions, the 1.5 mm and 2.0 mm laser-thermal-assisted balloon angioplasty devices were approved by the United States FDA in March 1987, for iliac and distal artery lesions. This approval was based on the initial angiographic and clinical results (155 [71%] of 219 attempted lesions), with the lesions subjectively categorized by the angiographer into those considered possible or impossible to treat by conventional balloon angioplasty. Table 5.3 details the overall initial clinical results in these cases.

Table 5.4 summarizes the one-year follow up data in 129 of the femoropopliteal lesions, from two of the centres (Boston University, USA, and Northern General Hospital, Sheffield, UK), compared to representative reports of patency for balloon angioplasty.

These initial studies showed that the combined laser-thermal balloon angioplasty technique was applicable in a higher percentage of cases, and that it would recanalize a higher percentage of long segment occlusions compared to balloon angioplasty alone. The rate of complications such as vessel perforations, groin haematomas, etc. was about 6–10%, and the incidence decreased following a rather severe 'learning curve' which occurred in almost all institutions.

Table 5.3 Initial angiographic and clinical results

Angioplasty category	N	Mean lesion length (cm)	Angiographic success		Clinical success	
			No.	%	No.	%
Possible	149	6.8	128	86	116	78
Stenosis	41		40	98	39	95
Occlusions	108		88	81	77	71
Impossible	70	11.7	44	63	39	56
Stenosis	4		4	100	4	100
Occlusions	66		40	61	35	53
Total	219	8.3	172	79	155	71

From Sanborn *et al.* (1989) with permission.

Table 5.4 Comparison of 1-year patency rates

Technique	Stenoses	Occlusions		
		3 cm	4–7 cm	7 cm
Laser-assisted balloon angioplasty	95	93	76	58
Balloon angioplasty alone				
Hewes *et al.*	81*	67*	82*	68*
Murray *et al.*	72*	86†		
Krepel *et al.*	80	93	50 (3 cm)	

Note: values are expressed as percentages.
*Redilatation rate of 12–20% was not considered recurrence.
†Value for all occlusions.
From Sanborn *et al.* (1989) with permission.

As a result of the initial reported success rapid development of laser devices continued, with an emphasis on increasing the size of the initial channel created by the probes and combining the thermal approach with controlled release of laser energy. The 2.5 mm, 3.5 mm and 5.0 mm diameter versions of a metal 'hot tip' device are shown in Fig. 5.31. The 2.5 mm probe was approved for use in October 1987, and represents one of the most popular probes that came into use following FDA approval of the laser-thermal technology.

A schematic representation of the 'hybrid' probe, approved in March 1989 for iliac and distal artery lesions, is given in Fig. 5.32; Fig. 5.33 demonstrates the emission of argon energy from the tip of this device. The concept in the hybrid probe was to provide better forward ablation of tissue by partial emission (approximately 20%) of the 'free' laser energy combined with the metal-tip thermal effect.

Concomitant efforts by other manufacturers addressed additional methods of obtaining directed delivery of laser energy to the tissue interface; Fig. 5.34 demonstrates the concept of delivery via sapphire tips (Surgical Laser Technology, SLT) of various configurations. The contact probes produce tissue ablation by delivery of the laser energy in a configuration determined by the shape of the lens.

Rapid evolution of laser-thermal devices and introduction of controlled energy emission via the 'hybrid' concept or Spectraprobe (Trimedyne, Inc., Tustin, CA, USA) have led to the use of multiple probes, guidewires, etc.

Recanalization of a femoropopliteal occlusion using several devices is shown in Fig. 5.35.

The second laser system to receive the United States FDA approval delivers argon laser energy via a fibre which is coaxially aligned within the vessel by a balloon catheter (Lastac, GV Medical, Minneapolis, MN, USA; Fig. 5.36).

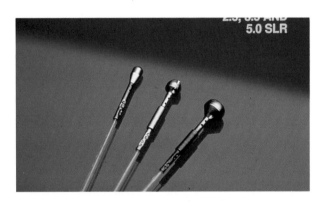

Fig. 5.31 Metal 'hot tip' device: 2.5 mm, 3.5 mm and 5.0 mm diameter versions.

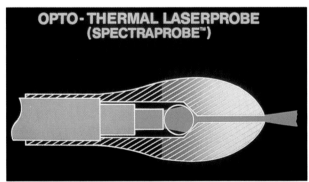

Fig. 5.32 'Hybrid' probe for iliac and distal artery lesions.

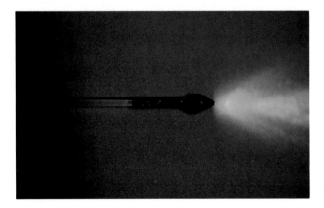

Fig. 5.33 Emission of argon energy from the tip of the 'hybrid' probe.

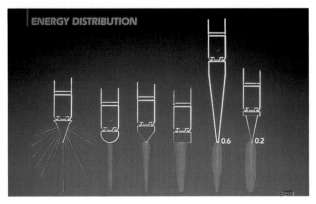

Fig. 5.34 Delivery of laser energy to tissue interface via sapphire tips.

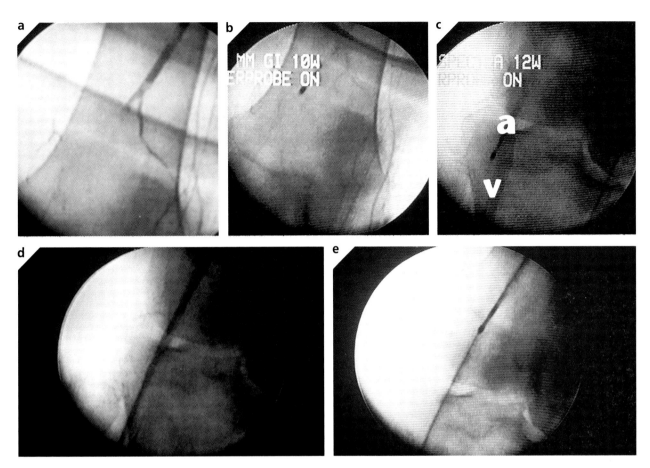

Fig. 5.35 Recanalization of obstructed femoral and popliteal arteries using different laser probe systems sequentially in one patient. (a) Femoral artery obstruction. **(b)** A 2.5 mm metal-tipped laser probe (arrow) tunnels through the obstruction located above the knee. **(c)** A 2.5 mm 'hybrid' probe, with 12 W of argon laser energy emitted through the end of the tip of the metal cap, is used to recanalize the artery behind the knee in an area that resisted passage of the 2.5 solid-capped thermal probe. Artery (a) overlying the vein (V) is visualized with contrast material from prior angiograms during the procedure. **(d)** Following recanalization of the artery, a 0.32 mm guidewire is passed. **(e)** A 2.5 mm solid-tipped Flex thermal probe is guided over the wire to enlarge the lumen.

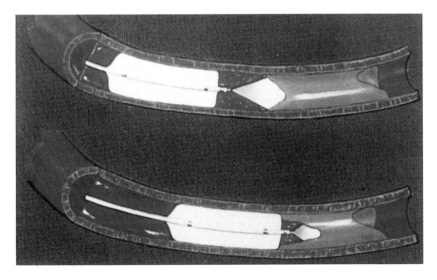

Fig. 5.36 Lastac argon laser system located in a vessel. The laser fibre is centred within the vessel lumen by a balloon (top); the catheter is advanced through the lesion and dilates any residual stenosis (bottom).

An additional system which has demonstrated significant clinical potential for treatment of both peripheral and coronary lesions is the excimer laser. This high energy, pulsed ultraviolet device has been extensively evaluated by several manufacturers (including Vaser, Inc., Indianapolis, IN, USA; Spectrametrics, Colorado Springs, CO, USA, Technolas Laser Technik, Munich, FRG; AIS, Irvine, CA, USA). The AIS laser has been the most widely investigated device and serves as a prototype for the potential of this instrument. Precise tissue ablation with minimal thermal or shock wave damage to surrounding tissue is pos-

sible if the laser parameters and delivery systems are chosen correctly (Figs 5.37 and 5.38).

Developmental problems relating to production of the excimer laser and delivery of energy through fibreoptics have now been resolved (Figs 5.39 and 5.40). Peripheral vascular stenoses and occlusions, as well as coronary stenoses, have been successfully treated with the excimer systems. One advantage of this device is its ability to recanalize calcified lesions which are not amenable to low energy thermal or continuous wave energy systems. The success of this controlled, free energy laser device has led to the develop-

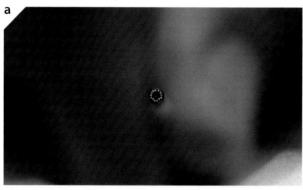

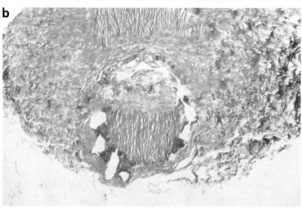

Fig. 5.37 Excimer laser system in operation. (a) Radially arranged fibres at the tip of a catheter delivering 208 nm excimer laser energy (10 Hz, 22 sec, 233 pulses, 30 mJ/mm^2 with 50 g pressure) to a fresh specimen of canine femoral artery (**b**). LM, ×40, trichrome stain. (Spectranetics excimer laser courtesy of Dr Diethrich, Arizona Heart Institute.)

Fig. 5.38 Precise incisions of fresh canine femoral artery. Excimer laser energy of 308 nm (10 Hz, 50 pulses, 40 mJ/mm^2) via a 600 μm fibre was used. Note minimal adjacent vacuolization of the arterial wall. LM, ×4, trichrome stain. (Spectranetics excimer laser courtesy of Dr Diethrich, Arizona Heart Institute.)

ment of a new generation of laser angioplasty systems which will improve the management of peripheral and coronary atherosclerotic disease.

Any contemporary discussion of endovascular surgical procedures and devices includes a consideration of the problems relating to guidance of angioplasty instruments and restenosis subsequent to initial recanalization. The guidance issue is particularly relevant, since the site of most atherosclerotic lesions is eccentric (see Chapter 1). For this reason, major emphasis is being directed towards the development of precise guidance methods for endoluminal instruments.

Several interesting laser devices are being developed and tested to address the guidance issue. Target-specific laser angioplasty may become possible by analysis of the emitted fluorescent patterns (laser-induced fluorescence) from the vessel wall (see Fig. 5.25, page 53). The MCM smart laser (formerly MCM Laboratories) used a dual catheter system controlled by a computer: a low power, 325 nm-induced fluorescence signal from the vessel wall was used to discriminate normal tissue from atherosclerotic lesions. As soon as the computer recognized the unique spectroscopic pattern of atheroma, it triggered a 480 nm high power, pulsed dye laser to ablate the atheroma (Fig. 5.41).

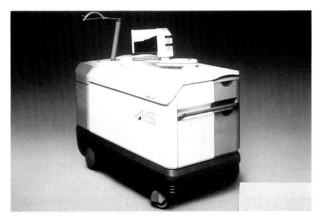

Fig. 5.39 Xenon chloride excimer laser. (From White and Grundfest, 1989, with permission.)

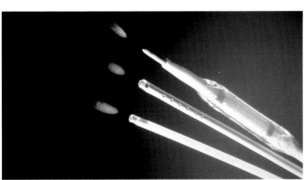

Fig. 5.40 New AIS excimer laser delivery systems under evaluation. Upper: A specially designed, large lumen 7F balloon angioplasty catheter. A central lumen accommodates a laser fibre. The middle catheter consists of 7 × 300 μm fibres arranged circumferentially around a 0.018 inch guidewire. This system permits distal dye injection and ablates a 2.2 mm channel. Lower: A highly flexible 12 fibre design for coronary applications. (From White and Grundfest, 1989, with permission.)

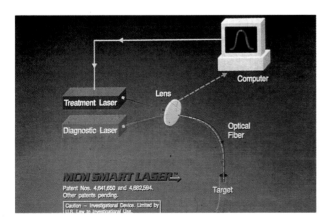

Fig. 5.41 MCM Smart Laser System. (From Murphy-Chutorian, 1989, with permission.)

An additional intriguing concept using spectroscopic guidance for controlled activation of a multifibre catheter, has been developed and evaluated by a collaborative effort of investigators from the Massachusetts Institute of Technology, Boston, and the Cleveland Clinic, Cleveland, USA (Figs 5.42–5.44).

Using argon laser radiation to excite both normal and atherosclerotic vessels, distinct patterns of fluorescence from each tissue can be disseminated from the 19-fibre array of multichannel spectral analyser. The potential for real-time imaging, using computer-processed 19-pixel spectroscopic images produced from fresh cadaver artery in vitro, is shown in Fig. 5.44. The spectra and images were produced by placing segments of normal and arteriosclerotic arteries side by side in a petri dish, and immersing them in blood. Images were obtained from tissue contact with the probe. Fluorescence from blood is minimal.

Another concept for achieving precise recanalization of the arterial lumen has been advanced by Medilase (Minneapolis, MN, USA). A motorized catheter positioner, operated by a computer 'touch-pad', directs a 480 nm pulsed dye laser to tissue ablation. The multilumen catheter incorporates the angioscope, balloon occlusion channel and irrigating lumen. This device is currently

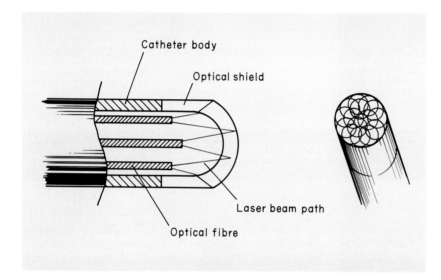

Fig. 5.42 Multifibre laser catheter. Left: Cross-sectional diagram showing an optical shield. Three fibres are depicted, along with the laser beam path of each. Note that the beams must be arranged so that light covers the entire surface of the shield. Right: Schematic representation of the intensity profiles of the laser light spots produced by 19 fibres in a 2.5 mm diameter device. (From Cothern et al., 1986, with permission.)

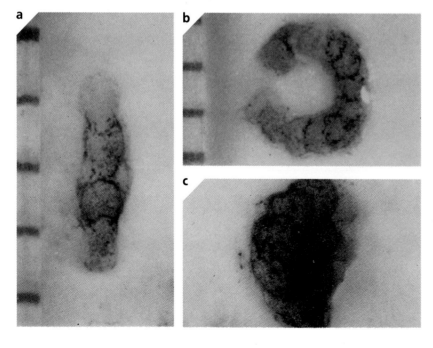

Fig. 5.43 Selective removal of plaque using the multifibre device. Composite holes were produced by firing selected fibres in the 19 fibre array. (**a**): Line. (**b**): Annulus. (**c**): Semicircle. Scale divisions are in millimetres. (From Cothern et al., with permission.)

being investigated for controlled tissue ablation, as depicted in Fig. 5.45.

Other new prototype delivery systems for laser devices, such as those described above, incorporate multiple modalities; i.e. spectroscopy, angioscopy in order to enhance the precision of initial vessel recanalizations. Of these, intravascular ultrasound is the most promising as a user-friendly and accurate way to accomplish the initial, precise, three-dimensional recanalization of occluded vessels (see page 10). This technology can be easily accommodated at the tip of 3–8F catheters, producing a detailed image of the thickness of the blood vessel wall. A prototype catheter incorporating an ultrasound transducer, which will be used in the newer devices to direct laser energy at the desired lesions for selective ablation, is shown in Fig. 5.46.

It has already been mentioned that restenosis of recanalized lesions remains the most serious drawback limiting the effectiveness of endoluminal surgery devices, particularly as the issue of guidance of devices in precise direction is resolved. Minimal progress has been made in defining the aetiology or control of restenosis.

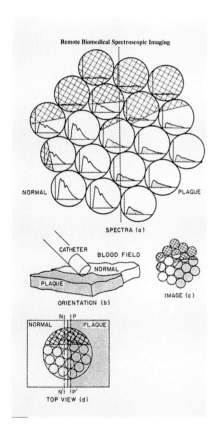

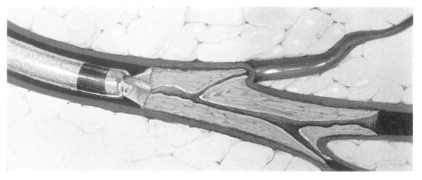

Fig. 5.45 Multilumen catheter used for controlled tissue ablation. (Courtesy of Medilase Inc., Minneapolis, MN, USA.)

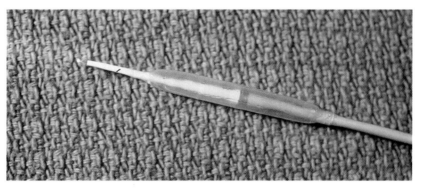

Fig. 5.44 Computer-processed images of test tissue configuration. (a) Spectra. **(b)** Geometry employed. **(c)** Laser spectroscope image. **(d)** A section diagram. The N–N′ section indicates normal tissue with a somewhat thickened intima; the P–P′ section indicates the presence of an early atherosclerotic lesion. (From Hoyt et al., with permission.)

Fig. 5.46 Phase array ultrasound transducer (gold ring) positioned in the centre of an angioplasty balloon catheter. A 200 μm laser fibre (emitting blue-green argon laser light) is passed through the central lumen of the catheter, to accomplish initial recanalization of the lumen. (Prototype ultrasound catheter courtesy of Endosonics Inc., Rancho Cucamonga, CA, USA.)

Spears has proposed an entirely different strategy in performing non-ablative Nd:YAG laser-heated balloon angioplasty. He suggested that low power Nd:YAG radiation could thermally seal plaque fissures in the artery wall produced by balloon dilatation, thus limiting elastic tissue recoil and hopefully preventing the incidence (approximately 5%) of abrupt vessel reclosure following angioplasty (Figs 5.47 and 5.48). The effect of the Spears Laser Balloon Angioplasty catheter (USCI, division of CR Bard, Bellerica, MA, USA) on artery 'recoil', plaque formation and restenosis is being investigated.

UTILITY, INDICATIONS AND LIMITATIONS OF LASER ANGIOPLASTY

Initial feasibility studies and successful reports of the use of laser thermal and controlled free energy devices were performed primarily by cardiologists and radiologists in stenotic lesions or short occlusions. These cases were chosen to compare the method to conventional balloon angioplasty and to enable evaluation of safety and efficacy of the technology in a low-risk patient population. These lesions usually do not cause either severe claudication or limb threat, the surgically accepted criterion for intervention, so that participation in the preliminary studies by surgeons was minimal. Later on, when surgeons and radiologists began to use these devices in longer occlusions in patients with conventional indica-

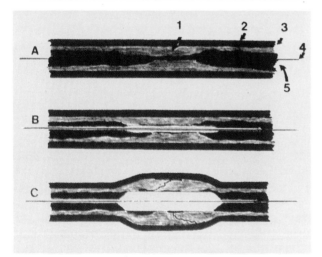

Fig. 5.47 Laser balloon angioplasty catheter.

Fig. 5.48A–C Conventional balloon angioplasty compared with laser balloon angioplasty. In the conventional procedure, a guidewire (4) is inserted into the arterial lumen (5). The balloon is threaded over the guidewire to the obstructing plaque (1) and inflated, sometimes causing dissection of the arterial wall to the media (3), or occasionally over the adventitia (2).

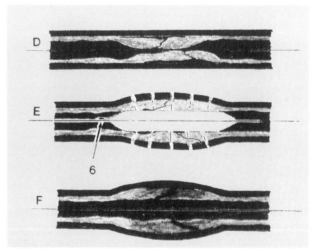

Fig. 5.48D–F Extensive dissection may cause abrupt reclosure (**D**). In this instance, laser balloon angioplasty (**E**) may be useful in fusing dissected layers of arterial wall, resulting in a smooth, dilated lumen (**F**). Lasing complications may be avoided by using an acoustic sensor (6) to detect the onset of tissue vapourization. (From Hichle et al., 1985, with permission.)

tions for surgery, the incidence of arterial wall perforations, reocclusion and early restenosis increased dramatically. This finding, coupled with the rapid evolution of technology, consumer and media interest, multiple subspecialty application (cardiologists, radiologists and surgeons) for different indications, together with a significant economic impetus for use and development, made laser angioplasty a highly controversial issue.

At present, it is reasonable to state that laser angioplasty is an investigational method which is undergoing rapid evolution, and that current success is inferior to conventional surgical methods, with the exception of limited applications which will be described in the following case presentations. An overall estimate of the utility of laser angioplasty with regard to length and site of occlusion is presented in Tables 5.5 and 5.6.

Analysis of these data and a review of the cases which have been managed in this way suggest that indications for using laser angioplasty may include:

1 Arterial stenosis and short occlusions.

2 Iliac lesions.

3 Chronically occluded PTFE grafts.

4 Selected patients who are at high risk for conventional surgery but where an interval patency may improve the operability at a later date.

Table 5.5 Estimated success rates related to length of lesion*		
	Initial recanalization	Follow-up patency
Stenoses	>95%	80%
1–3 cm	85–90%	60–70%
3–7 cm	75%	50–60%
7–10 cm	65%	45%
>10 cm	55%	20–40%

*Values estimated from survey of the currently available values (published and unpublished data) at 12–18 months follow-up.
From White & White (1989a) with permission.

Table 5.6 Success rates related to site of lesion			
	Initial success	Follow-up patency	
Iliac	80%	70%	Stenosis 80%
			Occlusion 50%
Mid-SFA	70%	60%	Stenosis 70%
			Occlusion 50%
Diffuse SFA	50–60%	40%	
Distal pop.	50%	20%	

From White & White (1989a) with permission.

Criteria for choosing patients for laser angio-plasty should include conventional surgical indications, with the procedure performed by an experienced surgeon. One reason to be conservative when treating minimal disease with the current state-of-the-art devices is that short stenoses or occlusions can be converted to long occlusions, if an imprecise technique is used or complications occur (Fig. 5.49).

Additional complications, including bleeding into the retroperitoneum from a femoral artery puncture above the inguinal ligament or from a perforated intra-abdominal vessel, and unsuccess-ful procedures requiring further surgical intervention to overcome vascular insufficiency, are best accommodated in the operating room where expedient repair can be initiated.

Fig. 5.50 illustrates a particularly appealing application for laser recanalization. Occlusions of the iliac vessels can frequently be treated by retrograde femoral artery insertion of devices. This case is particularly instructive, as it highlights the lack of lesion debulking by current devices and stresses the need for improved removal of tissue by newer devices (Fig. 5.50c). The iliac artery reoccluded at ten months postoperatively, most

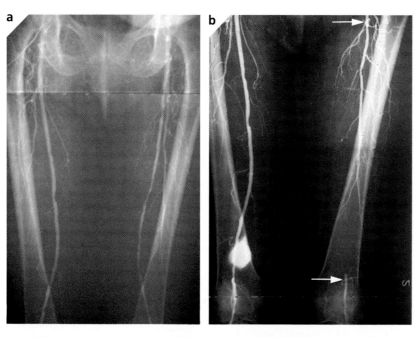

Fig. 5.49 Several discrete lesions in the superficial femoral artery. (a) These lesions in a 63-year-old female were easily treated with a laser thermal device over a guidewire. **(b)** Occlusion of the entire length of the superficial femoral artery (arrows) occurred two months following the procedure. (From White, 1990a, with permission.)

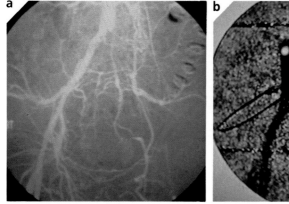
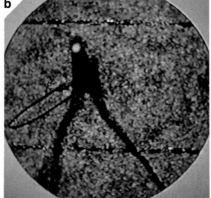
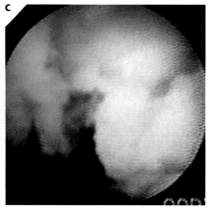

Fig. 5.50 Recanalization of a long occlusion of the left iliac artery. This procedure **(a)** is demonstrated by an image-enhanced angiogram of the vessel **(b)**, using laser thermal angioplasty.

(c) Angioscopic view of the intraluminal surface of the left iliac artery subsequent to recanalization, as visualized on the arteriogram in **(b)**. (From White et al., 1990b with permission.)

likely due to inadequate tissue removal at the initial procedure.

In a limited group of patients, veins are unsuitable for lower limb reconstruction, because they have been used in previous coronary or peripheral reconstructions, or are found to be inadequate by preoperative duplex examination or venography. Some patients in this category present with failed, chronically occluded PTFE prostheses which cannot be reopened by thrombectomy, as distal anastomotic hyperplasia has occluded the lumen and cannot be crossed by a guidewire. Furthermore, these lesions do not respond well to balloon angioplasty, because the inelastic prosthesis does not permit balloon dilatation and fracture of the lesion. In such cases, we have found that some chronically occluded PTFE prostheses can be easily recanalized by laser thermal devices, as the graft resists perforation and guides the probe through the intimal hyperplastic lesion (Figs 5.51 and 5.52).

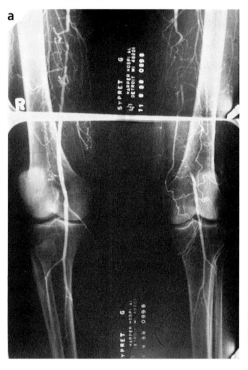
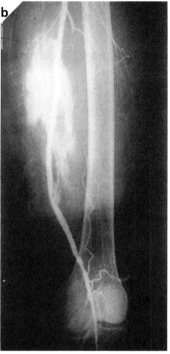

Fig. 5.51 Occlusion of the left superficial femoral artery and severe claudication. (a) Preoperative arteriogram of a 63-year-old female. A PTFE femoropopliteal bypass above the knee occluded five years previously. (b) Attempted recanalization of the superficial femoral artery by laser thermal angioplasty was unsuccessful (note extravasated dye in the thigh from arterial perforation), but the chronically occluded PTFE graft was easily reopened by thermal ablation of the distal anastomotic lesion which could not be crossed by a guidewire. The graft remains patent at 12 months following the procedure. (From White et al., 1990b, with permission.)

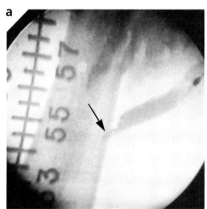
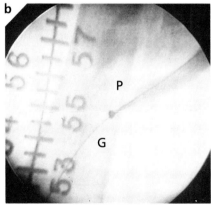
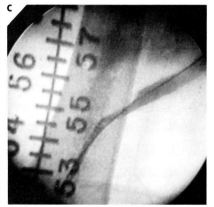

Fig. 5.52 Treatment of thrombosed PTFE prosthesis. (a) With residual obstruction at the graft-artery anastomosis (arrow), following removal of thrombus from the proximal segment. (b) Following recanalization of the obstruction with a 2.5 mm laser-thermal probe, a 3.5 mm probe (P) over a guidewire (G) enlarges the opening. (c) Restoration of flow remained for nine months before reocclusion occurred. (From White and White, 1989b, with permission.)

Another useful application of the laser angioplasty devices is in selected patients who are at high risk for conventional therapy or can benefit by an interval patency until definitive surgery can be performed (Fig. 5.53).

FUTURE DEVELOPMENTS

In summary, the initial results of laser angioplasty have been very promising for a technology which has only been evaluated for a five-year period since the preliminary studies were performed. Dramatic evolution is occurring in this highly controversial field, generating significant interest in physicians and lay public.

Future developments which are required if the technology is to survive are precise guidance of laser energy through the vessel lumen without perforation or surrounding tissue damage, and subsequent debulking of lesions to enhance short-term patency. Where restenosis does occur, close follow up – particularly with colour flow duplex scanning (see pages 134 and 135) and non-invasive haemodynamic testing – will enable serial percutaneous recanalization with 'over-the-wire' devices before reocclusion occurs. The ultimate final step in resolving the problem of recurrence rests on defining the aetiology and establishing methods that will arrest restenosis. The current dilemma regarding imprecise recanalization is exemplified in Fig. 5.54.

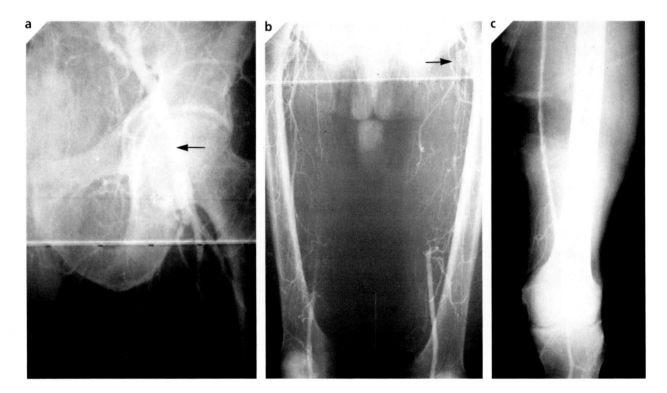

Fig. 5.53 Laser angioplasty in a high risk patient.
(a) and **(b)** Preoperative angiograms of a 72-year-old male with rest pain, ulcers over two toes and ankle/brachial ratio of 0.3 at eight weeks following myocardial infarction, with a left ventricular ejection function of 20%. The studies reveal discrete lesions of the common femoral artery (arrow), and **(b)** a 20 cm occlusion of the superficial femoral artery (arrows). Removal of the femoral artery plaque and laser-thermal recanalization of the superficial femoral artery **(c)** through a groin incision increased the ankle/brachial ratio to 0.8, with healing of the toes. The femoropopliteal repair has recently reoccluded, and the patient is undergoing elective bypass for claudication. (From White and White, 1989b, with permission.)

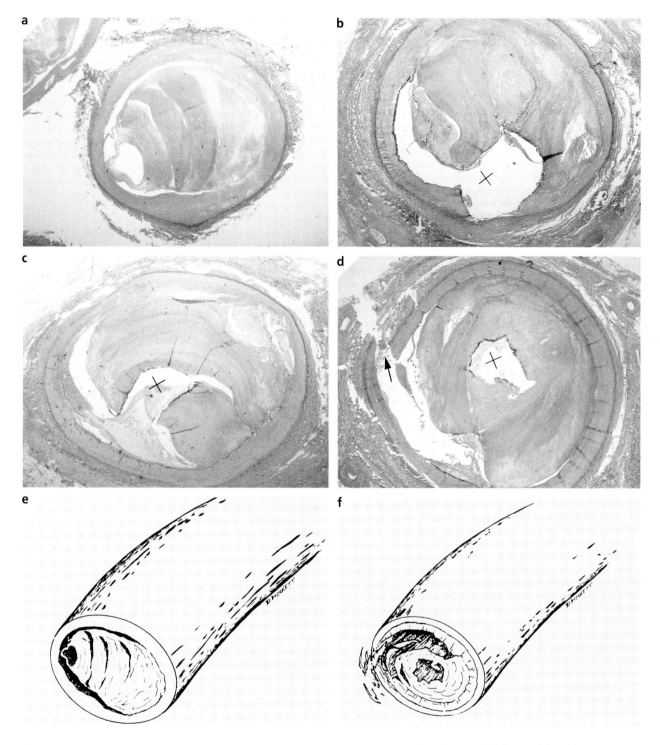

Fig. 5.54 Serial sections of the popliteal artery from a failed recanalization due to perforation. (a) Eccentric arterial occlusion distal to the perforation, identifying the site of the lesion. **(b)** and **(c)** Laser thermal channels (X) with associated balloon dilatation fractures in the plaques. **(d)** Arterial wall perforation at a site of combined laser-thermal probe and balloon dilatation disruption of the vessel wall (arrows). One passage of the thermal probe remained centrally (X). **(e)** Three-dimensional representation of the eccentric arterial lesion depicted in **(a)**. **(f)** Resulting perforation.

References

American National Standards Institute (1988) American National Standard For Safe Use of Lasers In Health Care Facilities, ANSI Standard 2-136.3, available from ANSI, 1430 Broadway, New York, NY 10018.

Cothern, R.M., Hayes, G.B., Kramer, J.R. *et al.* (1986) A multishield catheter with an optical shield for laser angiosurgery. *Lasers Life Sci.*, **1**, 1–12.

Cumberland, D.C., Sanborn, T.A., Tayler, D.I. *et al.* (1986) Percutaneous laser thermal angioplasty: initial results with a laser probe in total peripheral artery occlusions, *Lancet*, **i**, 1457–9.

Dixon, J.A. (ed.) (1987) *Surgical Applications of Lasers*, 2nd edn, Year Book Medical, Chicago.

Einstein, A. (1917) Zur quantem theorie dr strahlung. *Phys. Zect.*, **18**, 121.

Grundfest, W.S., Litvak, F., Glick, S. *et al.* (1987) Current status and future prospects for angioscopy and laser angioplasty. *J. Vasc. Surg.*, **5**, 667–2.

Grundfest, W.S. *et al.* (1989) Excimer laser angioplasty: recent development and clinical trials, in *Lasers in Cardiovascular Disease*, 2nd edn (eds R.A. White and W.S. Grundfest), Yearbook Medical, Chicago, pp. 130–40.

Hichle, J.F., Bourgelais, D.B., Shapstay, S. *et al.* (1985) *Am. J. Cardiol.*, **56**, 953–7.

Hoyt, C.C., Richards-Kortum, R.R., Costello, B. *et al.* (1988) Remote biomedical spectroscopic imaging of human artery wall. *Lasers Surg. Med.*, **8**, 1–9.

Isner, J.M. (1989) Blood, in *Cardiovascular Laser Therapy* (eds J.M. Isner and R. Clarke), Raven, New York., pp. 39–62.

Isner, J.M. (1989) Pathology, in *Cardiovascular Laser Therapy* (eds J.M. Isner and R. Clarke), Raven, New York, pp. 83–97.

Isner, J.M. and Clarke, R.H. (eds) (1989) *Cardiovascular Laser Therapy* Raven, New York.

Laser Safety Guide, Laser Institute of American 5151 Monroe Street, Toledo, Ohio 43623.

Leon, M.B., Lu, D.Y., Prevost, L.C. *et al.* (1988) Human arterial surface fluorescence: atherosclerotic plaque identification and effects of laser atheroma ablation. *J. Am. Coll. Cardiol.*, **12**, 92–102.

Murphy-Chutorian, D. (1989) Laser angioplasty and endarterecromy: present status and future potential, in *Current Critical Problems in Vascular Surgery* (ed. F. Veith), Quality Medical Publishing, St Louis, MO, pp. 188–94.

Sanborn, T.A. (ed.) (1989) *Laser Angioplasty*, Alan R. Liss, New York.

Sliney, D. (1985) Laser tissue interactions. *Clin. Chest Med.*, **6**, 203–8.

Steg, P.G. and Menasche, P. (1989) Utilization of laser arterial angioplasty. *Ann. Surg.*, **3**, 86–94.

White, R.A. (1988) in *Basic Physics of Laser Energy in Arterial Surgery: New Diagnostic and Operative Techniques* (eds J.J. Bergan and J.S.T. Yao), Grune & Stratton, Orlando, FL, pp. 33–44.

White, R.A. (1990a) The application of laser technology to vascular surgery. *Circulation*, in press.

White, R.A., White, G.H., Mehringer, C.M., *et al.* (1990b) A clinical trial of laser angioplasty in high-risk patients with advanced peripheral vascular disease. *Ann. Surg.*, in press.

White, R.A. and Grundfest, W.S. (eds) (1989) *Lasers in Cardiovascular Disease: Clinical Applications Alterative Angioplasty Devices and Guidance Systems*, 2nd edn, Year Book Medical, Chicago.

White, R.A. and White, G.H. (1989a) Laser thermal probe recanalization of occluded arteries. *J. Vasc. Surg.*, **9**, 598–608.

White, R.A. and White, G.H. (1989b) Laser angioplasty: development, current status and future perspectives. *Semin. Vasc. Surg.*, **2**, 123–42.

6 Atherectomy

MECHANICAL ATHERECTOMY BY INTRAVASCULAR DEVICES

The term 'atherectomy' is relatively new, and has come to signify the intravascular removal or debulking of atherosclerotic plaque by a variety of mechanical catheter devices.

Restenosis after conventional balloon angioplasty occurs in at least 30–40% of treated vessels, and is partly due to the fact that angioplasty dilates and remodels the lumen without removing the occlusive material from the vessel. In contrast, atherectomy devices are designed to physically remove plaque from the vessel; this is done in piecemeal fashion by cutting, drilling or pulverizing atheroma, thus producing a luminal surface quite different from open surgical endarterectomy.

Some of the currently available atherectomy devices are equipped with mechanisms for the extraction of fragments of ablated plaque. Other systems aim to reduce plaque to microparticles, which then circulate in the blood stream without producing clinically evident embolization. Atherectomy catheters are designed primarily for percutaneous use through an arterial sheath, but they may also be introduced via a small cutdown incision or as part of a conventional vascular surgical operation. Larger catheter sizes are more suited to intraoperative application.

Atherectomy may be the sole mode of therapy or used in conjunction with balloon dilatation. Most current devices are suitable only for stenotic lesions, and are inserted over a guidewire. If the stenotic arterial lumen is not sufficiently enlarged after a successful atherectomy procedure, adjunctive balloon dilatation is often performed. As a corollary, balloon angioplasty complications (particularly dissection or acute occlusion) or inadequate recanalization may be improved by subsequent passage of an atherectomy catheter.

Precise indications for atherectomy have not yet been defined; its true role in the management of vascular disease will be determined by further technological developments regarding instrumentation, as well as by extensive clinical experience. Although initial success has been achieved with the devices reported below, restenosis has been a problem, and the long term outcome of atherectomy in a diseased vessel is still unknown.

ATHERECTOMY DEVICES AND TECHNIQUES

The following are a series of illustrations (Figs 6.1–6.24) depicting various devices for atherectomy; the accompanying captions discuss their particular applications and the different atherectomy techniques. Fig. 6.1 shows an example of atherectomy application.

Fig. 6.1 An atherectomy device in use. This is introduced percutaneously via a 9F femoral artery sheath for treatment of a stenotic lesion of the distal superficial femoral artery. The catheter section of the device allows distal intravascular access of the mechanical tip, with control applied from the external motor drive unit.

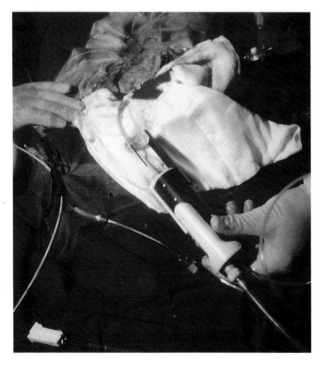

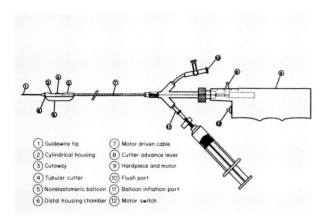

Fig. 6.2 The Simpson Atherocath. This consists of a catheter with a distal cutting blade and its housing chamber, including an attached positioning balloon. The proximal aspect of the catheter is coupled to a hand-held motor unit, and has two ports for fluid flush and balloon inflation. A lever on the motor drive unit is used to advance the rotating cutting blade into the distal chamber. The non-elastic balloon (5) pushes the cutaway (3) against the plaque. The tubular cutter (4) shaves a section of plaque and impacts it in the distal chamber (6). (From Chin and Fogarty, 1989, with permission.)

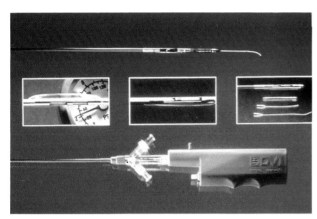

Fig. 6.3 The Simpson Atherocath. The distal housing unit is a cylinder with a longitudinal opening on one side and a balloon attached to the opposite wall. The cup-shaped cutting blade lies within the chamber, and may be rotated at speeds of up to 2000 r.p.m. by an attached cable driven by the motor unit. The balloon is opposite the window of the chamber, so that inflation pushes the atheroma into the chamber opening where it may be engaged by the cutting blade. A floppy guidewire is attached to the chamber and precedes it into the stenotic lesion. (Courtesy of Devices for Vascular Intervention Inc., Redwood City, CA, USA.)

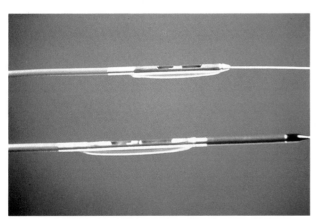

Fig. 6.4 Catheters for the peripheral vascular system. These range between 7–11F in diameter, with windows of 15 mm and 20 mm in length. Coronary artery designs are narrower (4.6–7F) and more flexible, with a window opening length of 10 mm. Excised atheromatous material is pushed by the blade into the distal containing section of the chamber so that it may be extracted by removal of the catheter. Early designs (top) had a small chamber that filled after only five or six blade passes. The more recent version has a larger chamber that will accommodate material from 20–25 cuts. (Courtesy of Devices for Vascular Intervention Inc., Redwood City, CA, USA.)

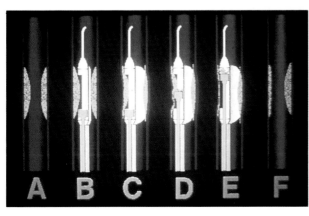

Fig. 6.5 Atherectomy technique. Atheromatous lesion (**A**) is defined by a preoperative angiogram. The catheter is advanced through the lesion, with the longitudinal window opening orientated towards the plaque (**B**). The balloon is inflated to 20–40 psi, to fix the plaque into the chamber (**C**). The motor is activated, and the rotating cutter is advanced through the engaged atheroma (**D**). The excised slice of tissue is pushed into the distal portion of the housing and trapped (**E**). Multiple passes of the cutter are usually required to smooth down and debulk the plaque. The balloon is deflated and the catheter removed to empty the chamber (**F**). (From Hinahara et al., 1989, with permission.)

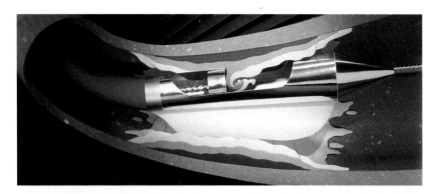

Fig. 6.6 Close up of the cutting process with the Simpson atherectomy catheter. (Courtesy of Devices for Vascular Intervention Inc., Redwood City, CA, USA.)

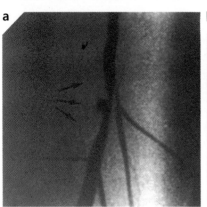
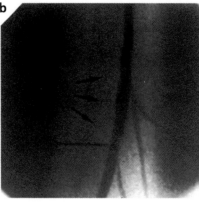
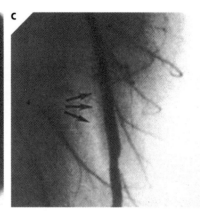

Fig. 6.7 Pre- and postatherectomy angiograms in a patient treated for stenosis of the superficial femoral artery. (a) An eccentric, ulcerated plaque is shown close to several branch vessels. This lesion had caused distal embolization. Such lesions are not well suited to balloon angioplasty, because of their eccentric distribution, length and complex composition with ulceration. Balloon dilatation may also compromise the adjacent branch offices. (b) Atherectomy resulted in restoration of a smooth, normal calibre artery. (c) A follow up angiogram at two years demonstrated continued patency of the treated area, with minimal restenosis.

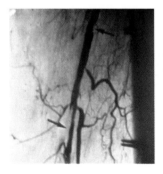
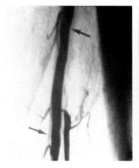
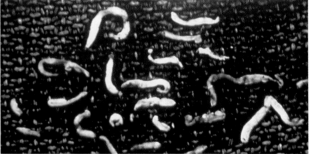

Fig. 6.8 Pre- and postatherectomy angiograms of a complex lesion in the superficial femoral artery. Excellent results can be seen after treatment. The atherectomy catheter was advanced percutaneously, via an arterial sheath in the common femoral artery, positioned at the site of the lesion to be treated, and held in position by inflation of the balloon during the cutting process. Tissue specimens are shown after removal from the distal chamber. Histological analysis of these fragments has revealed that lesions of restenosis following angioplasty consist primarily of an exuberant myointimal hyperplasia, with prominent smooth muscle cell proliferation covering the original atherosclerotic plaque. In contrast, de novo lesions usually consist of mature atherosclerotic plaque, often with regions of calcification, ulceration and organized thrombus over the surface. In the future, such biopsy specimens may prove helpful in determining the appropriate treatment, including drug therapy.

The **Simpson** atherectomy catheter, shown in Figs 6.2–6.9, may be indicated for extracting atheromatous tissue from stenotic plaques within peripheral and coronary arteries. Another indication may be the management of complications of balloon angioplasty, particularly dissection, intimal flap, inadequate recanalization and early restenosis. Adjunctive vascular stents may also be used in complex or recurrent lesions, particularly in the iliac or coronary arteries. Restenosis tends to occur rapidly if insufficient material is removed from the treated artery. If the residual lumen after treatment has under 30% stenosis, incidence of recurrent stenosis is approximately 25%.

Cordis Kensey atherectomy catheter system

This uses a different mechanism of action to debulk atheromatous plaque (Fig. 6.10). There is no cutting blade, but a rotating cam tip acts by pulverizing firm or fibrous atheromatous tissue into microparticles. The cam tip is rotated by a central drive shaft, housed within a flexible polyurethane catheter (Fig. 6.11). An external motor drive unit (Fig. 6.12) rotates the tip at speeds of up to 200 000 r.p.m., but rates of less than half this speed are now recommended.

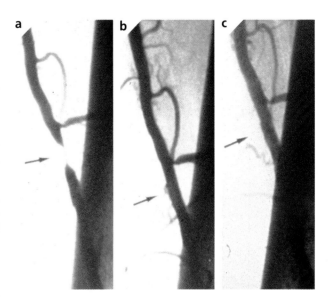

Fig. 6.9 Tight stenoses or total occlusions may need to be dilated with a balloon catheter, to allow the bulk of the atherectomy device to be passed through the lumen. In this case, a very tight stenosis in the adductor canal region of the superficial femoral artery (a) was successfully treated with atherectomy (b). The angiogram at six months follow up (c) shows no evidence of restenosis.

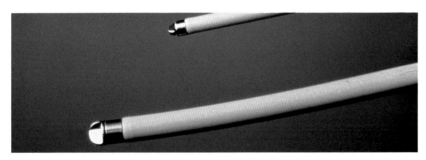

Fig. 6.10 The Cordis Kensey atherectomy catheter system. (Courtesy of Cordis Corporation, Miami, FL, USA.)

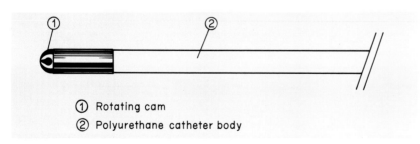

① Rotating cam
② Polyurethane catheter body

Fig. 6.11 The Kensey catheter and tip. Diagrammatic representation of the rotating cam at the tip which is housed in the polyurethane catheter body. (From Chin and Fogarty, 1989, with permission.)

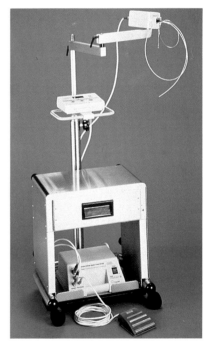

Fig. 6.12 External motor drive unit for the Kensey catheter. (Courtesy of Cordis Corporation, Miami, FL, USA.)

Within the catheter there is a coaxial lumen used for infusion of fluid. Fluid ejected from the rotating tip generates a radial jet which creates a vortex effect within the vessel, enhancing the emulsification of dislodged atherosclerotic debris (Figs 6.13 and 6.14). The fluid also serves to cool and lubricate the rotating cam.

Elastic tissue of the normal arterial wall is pushed aside and does not become damaged, whereas firm or fibrous atheroma is sculpted by the rotating tip and fluid jet.

There is no mechanism to remove fluid or microparticles from the vessel. Microembolized atheroma tissue seems to have little clinical effect. Access may be gained by a percutaneous sheath or intraoperative cutdown to the vessel. The fluid is usually injected at a rate of approximately 30 ml/min.

The catheter is typically advanced in a 'to-and-fro' fashion, with gentle and gradual progress down the vessel. A guidewire is not required, and the system is considered suitable for treatment of total occlusive lesions as well as arterial stenosis (Fig. 6.15).

Initial experience with this device was complicated by a fairly high rate of vessel perforation, since the catheter tends to follow the plane of least resistance which often takes it into the arterial wall. However, modifications of the instrument and increased experience with the technique have considerably reduced the incidence of this complication.

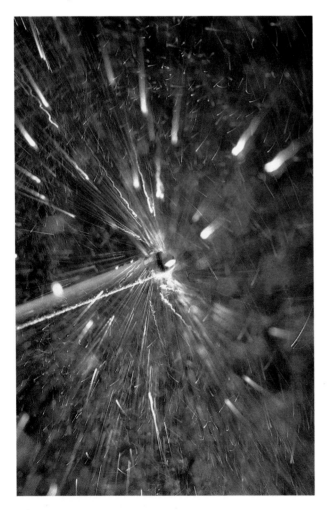

Fig. 6.13 Close up of the Kensey rotational atherectomy device. It demonstrates the radial fluid spray during activation. (Courtesy of Cordis Corporation, Miami, FL, USA.)

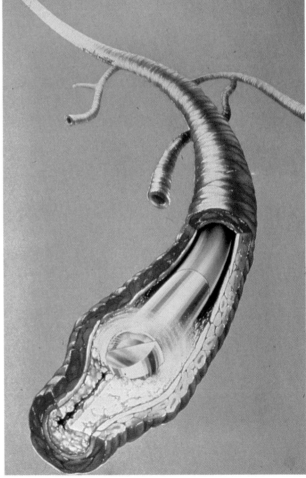

Fig. 6.14 Passage of a Kensey catheter through the arterial lumen. Diagrammatic representation; note the dilatation achieved by the cam action and spray of fluid emerging from the base of the cam assembly. (From Kensey, 1987, with permission.)

Auth rotablater atherectomy system

The Auth rotablater (Fig. 6.16) also consists of a rotating shaft which is used to drill out a core from the vessel lumen. The tip is a burr with its leading surface covered by metal-impregnated diamond chips (see Fig. 6.16). A flexible mechanical drive shaft, attached to the metal burr tip, is housed in a Teflon sheath inside the atherectomy catheter. The whole system is designed to be fed down the artery over a guidewire, and is essentially suitable for treatment of stenotic lesions. For total occlusions, a guidewire must first be passed through the lesion. The drive shaft is controlled by a turbine housed in a plastic casing attached to the proximal end of the catheter. Compressed air powers the turbine with a rota-

tion speed exceeding 100 000 r.p.m. (depending on the degree of pressure). The system also contains an irrigation port for infusion of fluid.

Different burrs that can be used with this device are illustrated in Fig. 6.17. The small size tips are designed for use in the peripheral vascular system, particularly the superficial femoral and popliteal arteries. The multiple diamond chips on the tip work as microknives, fracturing and fragmenting atheromatous plaque. A control knob on the motor drive casing allows the surgeon to advance or retract the burr tip over the guidewire. The drive shaft has a disengagement mechanism which prevents the artery from wrapping around the rotating burr or catheter at a low torque.

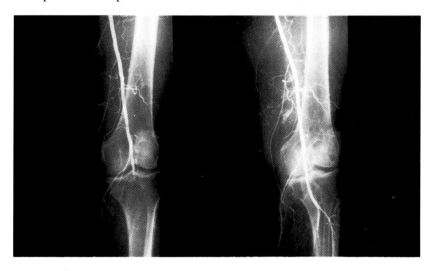

Fig. 6.15 Angiograms demonstrating the efficacy of the Kensey rotating tip atherectomy system. (Courtesy of Cordis Corporation, Miami, FL, USA.)

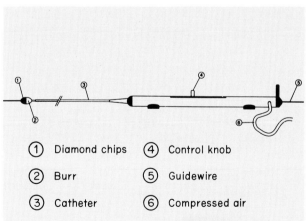

Fig. 6.16 The Auth rotablater atherectomy system. Diagrammatic representation of the mechanisms. (From Chin and Fogarty, 1989, with permission.)

① Diamond chips ④ Control knob
② Burr ⑤ Guidewire
③ Catheter ⑥ Compressed air

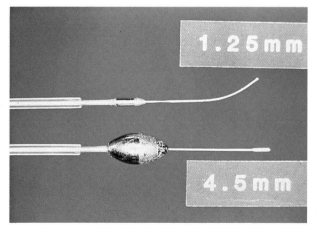

Fig. 6.17 Auth rotablater. Examples of burrs available with this device. (From Ahn et al., 1988, with permission.)

Animal experiments using labelled particles of atheroma have demonstrated that these particles are generally less than $1 \mu m$ in size, and pass through the small vessels of the leg accumulating in the lung, liver and reticular endothelial system.

Application of the Auth device results in a smooth intraluminal surface, without significant flaps or internal irregularities (Figs 6.18 and 6.19).

Transluminal extraction catheter (TEC)

The TEC atherectomy catheter (Fig. 6.20) also uses a rotating burr tip technique (Fig. 6.21). The tip has two very sharp blades which are used to cut plaque; the internal lumen of the hollow-tubed catheter is connected to suction, allowing extraction of the fragmented particles (Fig. 6.22). The procedure is performed over a guidewire and is suitable for stenotic lesions only.

The motor drive unit in clinical application is depicted in Fig. 6.23.

A clinical case, illustrated and discussed in Fig. 6.24a–f, highlights the technique and outcome of transluminal atherectomy.

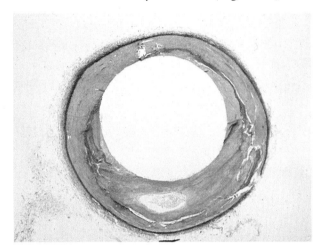

Fig. 6.18 Cross-section of an atherectomized artery from a cadaver. The results achieved with this technique are illustrated. (From Ahn et al., 1988, with permission.)

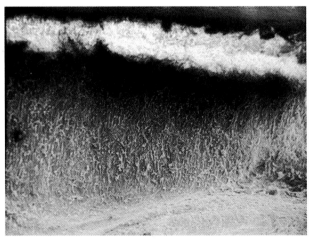

Fig. 6.19 Atherectomized popliteal artery, demonstrating a highly polished, smooth intimal surface. SEM, ×20. (From Ahn et al., 1988, with permission.)

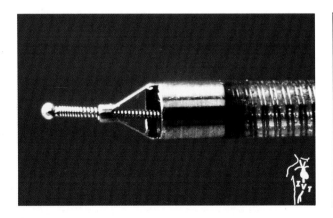

Fig. 6.20 The TEC atherectomy catheter. This uses a rotating burr tip technique. (Courtesy of Interventional Technologies Inc., San Diego, CA, USA.)

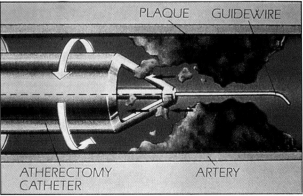

Fig. 6.21 Metallic blade tip of the TEC device. The blades rotate at 750 rpm. Fluid is infused through a separate lumen in the catheter, to irrigate the treated region and allow extraction of the particles with the fluid medium. (Courtesy of Interventional Technologies Inc., San Diego, CA, USA.)

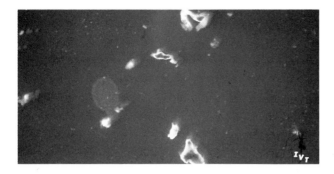

Fig. 6.22 Particles collected during a procedure with the transluminal extraction device. The size of such pieces of atheroma varies from microscopical to several millimetres. (Courtesy of Interventional Technologies Inc., San Diego, CA, USA.)

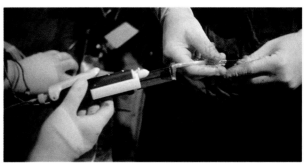

Fig. 6.23 Motor drive unit in clinical application. The atherectomy catheter segment is fed over a guidewire through a lumen in the motor drive unit, and is suitable for percutaneous or intraoperative application. Sequential use of larger sizes of catheter (5F, 7F and 9F) is recommended.

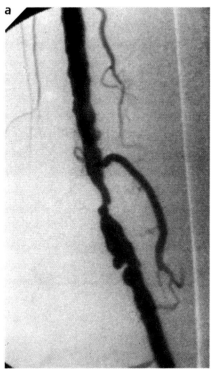

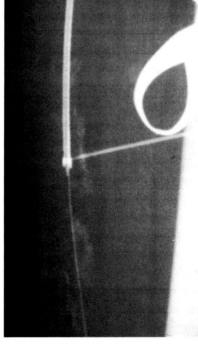

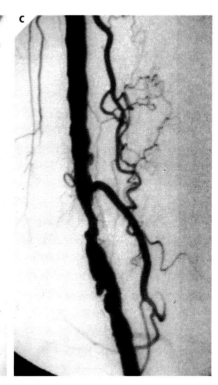

Fig. 6.24a Preoperative angiogram, showing multiple stenotic lesions within the superficial femoral artery. This patient had previously been treated with balloon angioplasty, with early recurrence of stenosis. The complex, ulcerated nature of these lesions suggests that repeat balloon angioplasty alone would not be the ideal management.

Fig. 6.24b Passage of the TEC atherectomy device over a guidewire down the artery. A radiological marker indicates the point of maximal stenosis. The catheter passed through this lesion with some difficulty, via a percutaneous sheath approach.

Fig. 6.24c Appearance of the treated artery immediately after passage of the atherectomy catheter. A wider lumen size is seen at the region of proximal stenosis. The distal lesion was not treated at this stage.

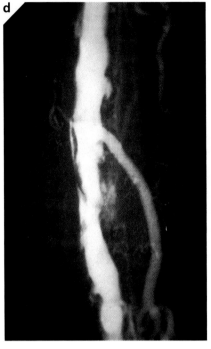

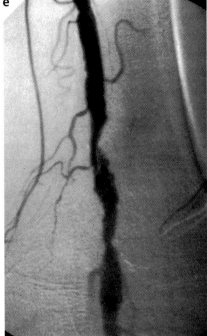

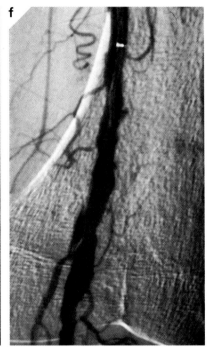

Fig. 6.24d Angiogram following adjunctive balloon dilatation. This shows widening of the vessel lumen, with angiographic appearance of wall dissection caused by the balloon. The clinical result was good, with return of the popliteal and distal pulses.

Fig. 6.24e Popliteal lesion in the same patient. The appearance of this distal lesion is also suggestive of complex plaque. Transluminal atherectomy was performed.

Fig. 6.24f Same artery following transluminal atherectomy and adjunctive balloon dilatation. A very satisfactory angiographic result is seen. Early restenosis of 15–30% at six months has been reported.

COMPLICATIONS

Complications of transluminal atherectomy are similar to those of other interventional techniques within the peripheral vascular system (see Fig. 6.25). The overall incidence should be less than 10%, with thrombosis and embolization being the most important complications.

In experienced hands, fewer than 5% of patients suffer complications; the long term systemic effects of microembolization have yet to be fully determined. Haemoglobinuria and haemolysis have been recorded on several occasions. Microembolization to distal tissues in the leg has not been a serious clinical problem, even though many particles must be embolized to the distal arterial beds.

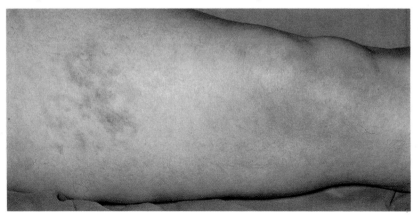

Fig. 6.25 Embolization to the skin over the superficial femoral artery. Such lesions have been seen with laser angioplasty and atherectomy procedures.

References

Ahn, S.S. (1989) Peripheral atherectomy. *Semin. Vasc. Surg.*, **2**, 143–54.

Ahn, S.S., Auth, D.C., Marcus, D.R. and Moore, W.S. (1988) Removal of focal atheromatous lesions by angioscopically guided high-speed rotary atherectomy: preliminary experimental observations. *J. Vasc. Surg.*, **7**, 292–300.

Chin, A.K. and Fogarty, T.J. (1989) Balloons and mechanical devices, in *Lasers in Cardiovascular Disease: Clinical Applications, Alternate Angioplasty Devices, and Guidance Systems* (eds R.A. White and W.S. Grundfest), Year Book Medical, Chicago, pp. 217–27.

Hinahara, T., Robertson, G.C., Selmon, M.R. *et al.* (1989) Percutaneous atherectomy: the Simpson atherectomy catheter, in *Endovascular Surgery* (eds W.S. Moore and S.S. Ahn), W.B. Saunders, Philadelphia, pp. 310–22.

Kensey, K.R., Nash, J.E., Abrahams, C. *et al.* (1987) Recanalization of obstructed arteries with a flexible, rotating catheter tip. *Radiology*, **165**, 387–9.

Simpson, J.B., Selmon, M.R., Robertson, G.C. *et al.* (1988) Transluminal atherectomy for occlusive peripheral vascular disease. *Am. J. Cardiol.*, **61**, 96G–101G.

Snyder, S.O., Wheeler, J.R., Gregory, R.T. *et al.* (1988) The Kensey Catheter: preliminary results with a transluminal atherectomy tool. *J. Vasc. Surg.*, **8**, 541–3.

Wholey, M.H. and Jarmolowski, C.R. (1989) New reperfusion devices: the Kensey catheter, the atherolytic reperfusion wire device, and the transluminal extraction catheter. *Radiology*, **172**, 947–52.

7 Intravascular Stents

Intravascular stents (i.e. endovascular splints) have been developed as a method to treat some of the inadequacies and complications of angio-plasty devices. At present, a variety of intravascular stents are being evaluated (Figs 7.1–7.5).

The proposed benefits of stents are seen in

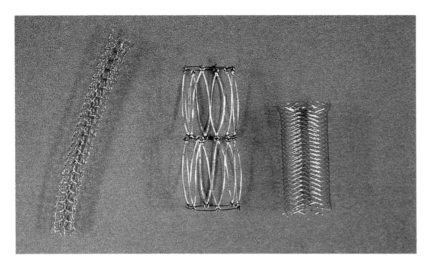

Fig. 7.1 Intravascular stents. Left: Strucker, a malleable tantalum stent. (Courtesy of Boston Scientific Corporation, Watertown, MA, USA) Centre: Gianturco, a self-expanding, stainless steel stent. (Courtesy of William Cook, Bloomington, IN, USA) Right: Medinvent, an expandable, stainless steel stent. (Courtesy of Pfizer, Minnetonka, MN, USA.) (From Wallace et al., 1989, with permission.)

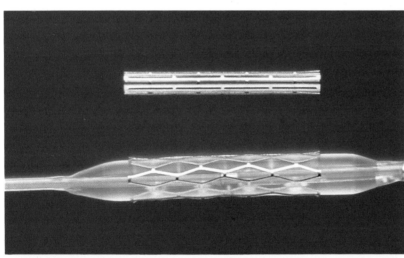

Fig. 7.2 Balloon-expandable Palmaz-Schatz stent. Top: The collapsed stent fits coaxially over a coronary angioplasty balloon catheter. Bottom: Inflation of the balloon results in the expansion of each rectangular slot into a diamond configuration.

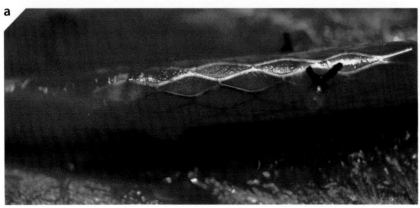

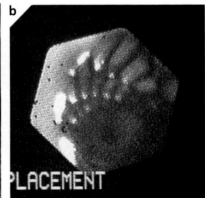

Fig. 7.3 Palmaz-Schatz stent. (a) Extraluminal appearance through the arterial wall. **(b)** Intraluminal angioscopic view.

relation to the treatment of acute reclosure of angioplasties from residual thrombotic material (flaps, dissections, etc.) or recoil of the vessel wall (Fig. 7.6). Furthermore, stents may be useful in preventing or retarding restenosis following recanalization.

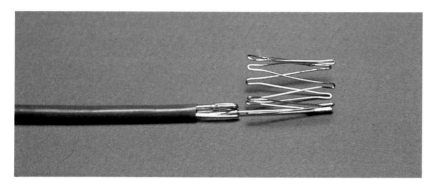

Fig. 7.4 Delivery of the Gianturco stent. A stiff wire is held against the stent as the outer sheath is withdrawn. (Courtesy of L. Machan, University of British Colombia, Canada.)

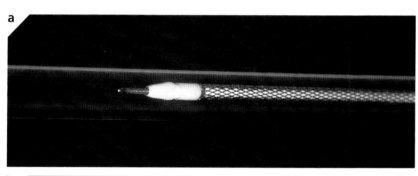

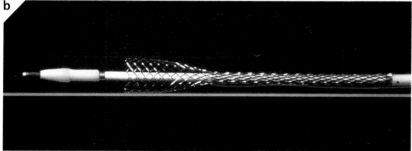

Fig. 7.5 Delivery of the Medinvent stent. (a) Prior to release. **(b)** The stent is released when a retractable hydraulic membrane is withdrawn. (Courtesy of L. Machan, University of British Columbia, Canada.)

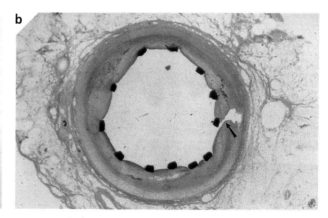

Fig. 7.6 Microphotographs of coronary artery from human cadaver. (a) Dilated but not stented coronary artery, with a typical intimal and medial dissection and lumen collapse. **(b)** Dilated and stented coronary artery, with a large intimal and medial tear 'tacked up' by stent struts (arrow). (From Schatz, 1989, with permission.)

Preliminary clinical evaluation of these devices has demonstrated their important role in salvaging patients with abrupt closure of coronary balloon angioplasties, by restoring patency and preventing myocardial infarctions. Similar benefits have been shown in the treatment of residual stenoses, flaps, dissections or recoil of large vessel angioplasties (Fig. 7.7).

Prevention of restenosis by stent therapy is yet to be demonstrated, therefore this particular application remains controversial, particularly since the risks of chronic thrombosis, dislodge-

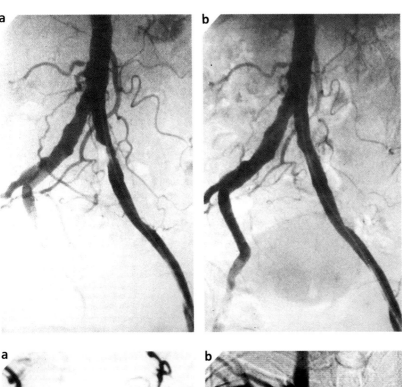

Fig. 7.7 Aortograms of left common iliac artery. (a) Residual stenosis due to recoil of a lesion following laser-assisted balloon angioplasty, with a residual pressure gradient of 20 mmHg. **(b)** Following insertion of a Palmaz-Schatz intravascular stent, showing total expansion of the artery and elimination of the pressure gradient. (Courtesy of E.B. Diethrich, Arizona Heart Institute, USA)

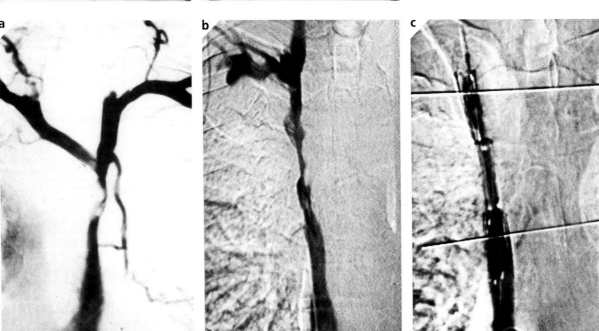

Fig. 7.8 Superior vena cava syndrome, secondary to bronchogenic carcinoma. (a) Superior vena cavagram following injection of contrast in each arm. A gradient of 40 mmHg was measured across the stenosis. **(b)** Selective injection via the right subclavian vein, prior to stent insertion. **(c)** Postinsertion of a Gianturco stent. Immediate clinical improvement was noted. (Courtesy of L. Machan, University of British Columbia, Canada.)

ment and migration or embolization are not insignificant with a rigid metal device. Further research and follow up studies are required before the use of intravascular stents is justified in this respect.

Additional promising areas for stent therapy are being evaluated, such as the expansion of major venous constrictions. Stenting of iliac veins and superior vena caval stenoses have been particularly appealing (Fig. 7.8), as has been the application of stent therapy in aneurysmal disease of the iliac artery (Fig. 7.9).

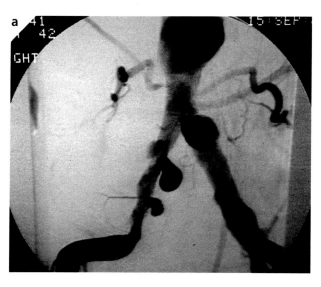 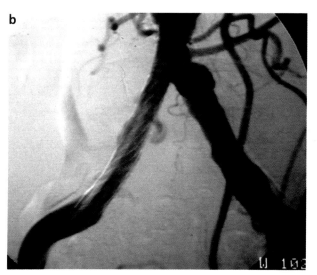

Fig. 7.9 Use of stents in aneurysmal disease of the iliac artery. (a) Multiple saccular aneurysms of the right iliac artery. **(b)** Expansion of the iliac artery lumen and obliteration of the aneurysms following stent placement.

References

Dichet P.A., Neville, R.F., Zwiebel, J.A., Freeman, S.M., Leon, M.B. and Anderson W.F. (1989) Seeding of intravascular stents with genetically engineered endothelial cells. *Circulation* 80, 1347–53.

Gunther, R.W., Vorwerk, D., Bohndorf, K., Peters, I., El-Din, A. and Messmer, B. (1989) Iliac and femoral artery stenoses and occlusions: treatment with intravascular stents. *Radiology* 726, 725–30.

King, S.B. (1989) Vascular stents and atherosclerosis. *Circulation* 79, 460–2.

Schatz, R. (1989) A view of vascular stents. *Circulation* 79, 445–57.

Sigwart, U., Puel, J., Mirkovitch, V., Joffre, F. and Kappenberger, L. (1987) Intravascular stents to prevent occlusion and restenosis after transluminal angioplasty. *New Eng. J. Med.* **316**, 701–6.

Sigwart, U., Urban, P., Golf, S., Kaufmann, U., Imbert, C., Fischer, A. and Kappenberger, L. (1988) Emergency stenting for acute occlusion after coronary balloon angioplasty. *Circulation* 78, 1121–7.

8 Additional Endovascular Techniques

THERMAL ABLATION DEVICES

Subsequent to the initial success of laser thermal devices, several more economical, non-laser thermal systems have been developed. The prototype device in this category is the radiofrequency (RF) generator (Advanced Interventional Systems Inc., Irvine, CA, USA), which operates at 50 MHz and delivers power up to 60 W. The gold-tipped catheters (Fig. 8.1) are energized by a battery power unit (Fig. 8.2); this provides a cost effective alternative to thermal devices.

Additional thermal systems (including electric and catalytic types) are also being developed and investigated (Figs 8.3–8.6), and may become alternatives to the RF device, if thermal ablation remains a viable modality.

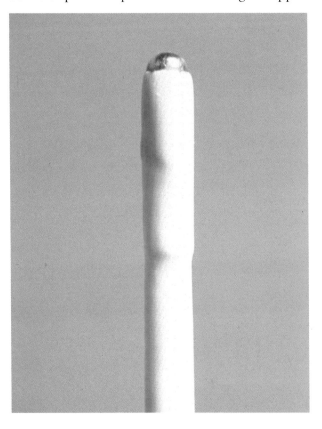

Fig. 8.1 Gold-tipped radiofrequency hot tip catheter. This features a high temperature plastic insulation that limits the shaft temperature to 90°. (From White and Grundfest, 1989, with permission.)

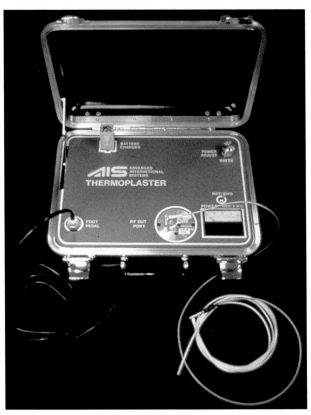

Fig. 8.2 Portable battery powered radiofrequency hot tip unit. (From White and Grundfest, 1989, with permission.)

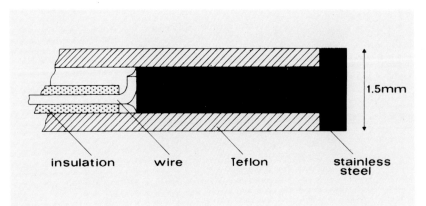

insulation   wire   Teflon   stainless steel

1.5mm

Fig. 8.3 Spark erosion electrode. Schematic representation. (From Slager et al., 1985, with permission.)

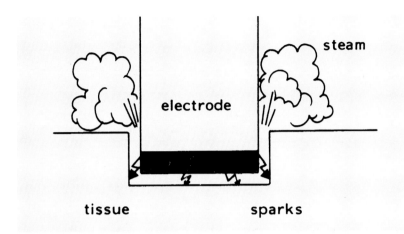

Fig. 8.4 Spark erosion process. Schematic representation: the steam layer isolates the electrode from the tissue. Sparks jumping between the electrode and tissue produce very high local energy densities that lead to tissue vapourization. (From Slager et al., 1985, with permission.)

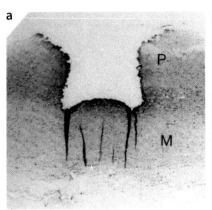 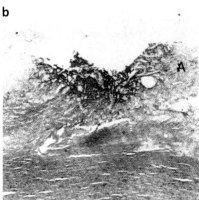 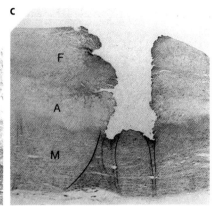

Fig. 8.5 Histological sections of aortic wall. (a) Section through the aortic wall showing a mainly fibrous plaque (P). Application of the spark erosion method, in a direction perpendicular to the area of the plaque, produced a punched-out crater extending to the superficial layers of the media (M). Two 10 msec pulses, each delivering approximately 1.7 J, produced this result. Note the very small dark rim representing the coagulation zone. H&E, ×28. **(b)** An atheromatous plaque with extensive lipid deposits (A). The crater created by the spark erosion technique was achieved with three 10 msec pulses, each delivering approximately 1.7 J. Note the frayed aspect of the border of the lesions, and thr broad dark coagulation zone. H&E, ×23. **(c)** Section through the aortic wall, with an atheromatous plaque (A) covered by a fibrous cap (F). The crater which extends to the superficial layers of the media (M) was achieved with four 10 msec pulses. Along the border of the crater, only a very small dark coagulation zone can be observed. H&E, ×27. (From Slager et al., 1985, with permission.)

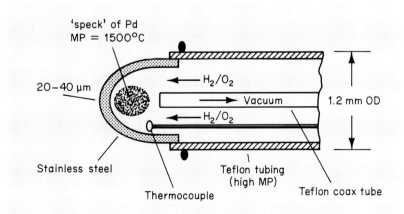

Fig. 8.6 Catalytic thermal tip catheter. Schematic representation, showing a palladium (Pd) sponge impregnated in the metallic tip and a double lumen catheter for gas delivery and water vapour evacuation. The device produces energy from hydrogen combustion. MP = melting point. (From Lu et al., 1989, with permission.)

ULTRASONIC TISSUE ABLATION

Ultrasonic ablation of atherosclerotic plaques has been evaluated as a method of removing abnormal tissues while preserving normal arterial wall. Pulsed and continuous energy is delivered to plaques via a wire probe (Fig. 8.7), with histological evidence of ablation which conforms to the shape of the probe tip (Fig. 8.8). By modifying the duration, mode and magnitude of power output, pulsed energy has been shown to limit thermal perforations, and to provide preliminary *in vivo* ablation of chronic fibrocellular occlusions in canine femoral arteries (Fig. 8.9).

WATER JET PLAQUE DISSOLUTION

A method for plaque dissolution has been identified which percutaneously delivers a pulsatile high velocity stream of saline to the site of atheromatous lesion within a coronary or peripheral artery. A prototype rheolytic guidewire (Fig. 8.10), capable of delivering 30 000 psi of internal pressure, was designed to fit within the guidewire lumen of a standard PTCA catheter.

INTRALUMINAL SURGICAL INSTRUMENTS

Subsequent to the development of angioscopy to improve guidance of intravascular instruments and visually evaluate the outcome of vascular interventions, many devices have evolved which incorporate the new technologies to enhance intraluminal procedures. The Fogarty-Chin valvulotome is an example of a miniaturized instrument for visually guided disruption of *in situ* vein valve cusps (Fig. 8.11). Intraluminal instruments which are being investigated for specialized intravascular applications are demonstrated in Fig. 8.12. In the future, these new techniques may be used to improve the guidance and use of other older vascular methods, such as gas endarterectomy, and devices including ring strippers and biopsy forceps.

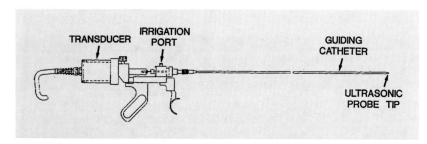

Fig. 8.7 Ultrasonic device used for arterial plaque ablation. Schematic representation: the ultrasound transducer is connected to a wire probe, which is ensheathed in an angiographic catheter. (From Siegel et al., 1988, with permission.)

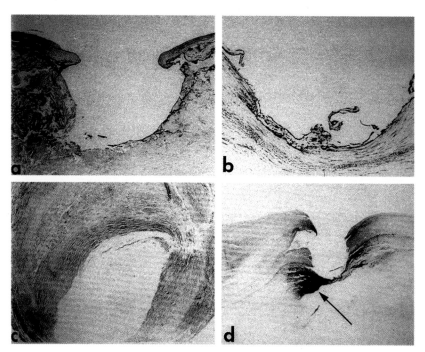

Fig. 8.8 Examples of results with the solid wire ultrasound probe. (a) Distinct crater limited to intimal plaque after application of the probe perpendicularly to the intimal surface. H&E, ×40. **(b)** Similar application, but here the crater extends into the arterial media. H&E, ×40. **(c)** Recanalized vessel which was completely occluded prior to application of the ultrasound probe. H&E, ×4. [In **(b)** and **(c)**, the black material lining the craters is India ink which was added to the site of application for later identification.] **(d)** Perforated vessel with a defect through the intima and media into the adventitia, showing thermal injury. H&E, ×40. (From Siegel et al., 1988, with permission.)

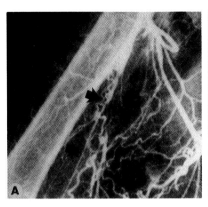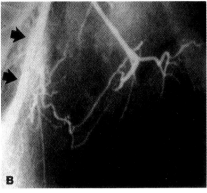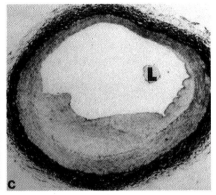

Fig. 8.9 *In vivo* recanalization of a chronic (12 month) fibrocellular occlusion in canine femoral artery. (a) Prior to ultrasound, a long and severely narrowed right femoral artery is present in association with extensive collateral vessels. (b) After intra-arterial ultrasonic recanalization, the lumen is markedly enlarged and the collateral vessels are no longer evident. (c) Histological section of the recanalized vessel demonstrates a mild, residual, fibrous, eccentric stenosis (L = lumen). H&E, ×40. (From Siegel et al., 1988, with permission.)

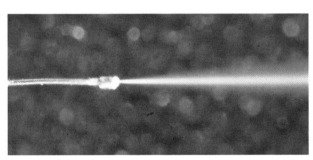

Fig. 8.10 Pulsatile high velocity water for plaque dissolution. The ability of rheolytic devices to cut through calcified and soft lesions without thermal damage and with small particulate effluent (2–15 μm for fresh human plaque), may offer an advantage over other atherectomy methods. The flexibility of this guidewire suggests that it may have applications in small vessels. (Courtesy of W Drasler and R Dutcher, Possis Medical, Inc., Minneapolis, MN, USA.)

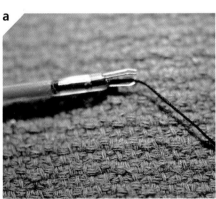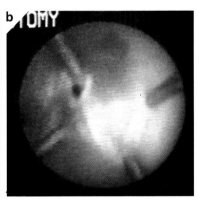

Fig. 8.11 Fogarty-Chin valvulotome. (a) This device combines a four-pronged metal valvulotomy device with an angioscope, and is guided over a suture which is passed through the lumen. (b) Angioscopic view of the valvulotomy device incising valve cusps.

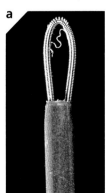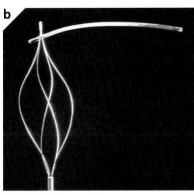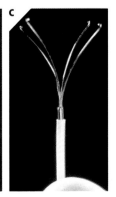

Fig. 8.12a,b,c Examples of intraluminal instruments. These are being investigated for specialized intravascular applications.

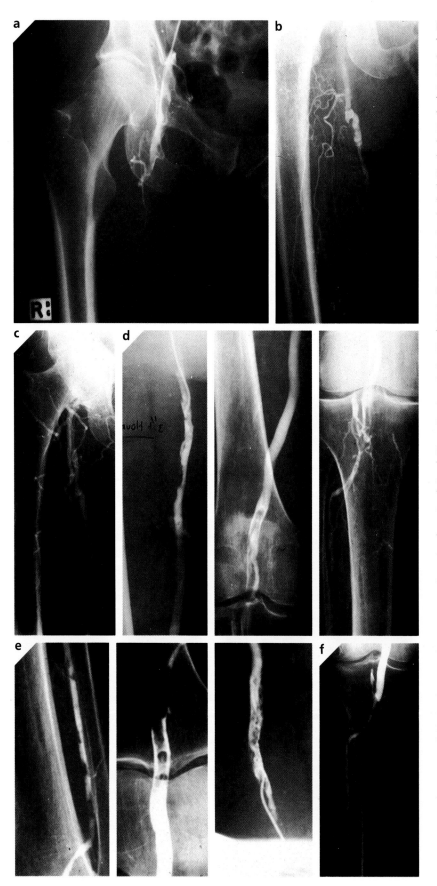

Fig. 8.13a–f Regional thrombolytic infusion of occluded femoropopliteal bypass graft. (a) The initial angiogram reveals thrombus in the common femoral artery, with non-visualization of the bypass graft or the profunda femoris artery. Since the leg was viable, a regional infusion of streptokinase was commenced via the angiographic catheter which had been introduced from the contralateral femoral approach. (b) Following several hours of infusion, the common femoral artery has been cleared of thrombus, with opening of several small collateral branches and the proximal 5 cm of the bypass graft. Partially lysed thrombus is seen near the proximal anastomosis. (c) After 3.5 hours of infusion, the small collateral branches around the hip are better defined, and a further segment of the bypass graft is now recanalized. A localized stenosis, or kink, is seen several centimetres from the graft origin. (d) The angiogram now reveals filling of the distal graft, and some filling of the runoff below the knee. Filling defects are seen within the graft, representing undissolved thrombus. (e) The infusion catheter is fed further down into the thrombus; after 12 hours of infusion, more localized thrombus or embolic material is seen within the distal portions of the graft, and within the anterior tibial artery, which is the primary run-off vessel. (f) Following 24 hours of infusion, the graft has now been cleared of all residual thrombus, and the segments of thrombus within the anterior tibial artery have been lysed. At this time, the popliteal and dorsalis pedis pulses were present. The patient was maintained on heparin infusion for a further 48 hours.

THROMBOLYTIC THERAPY

Thrombolytic therapy involves the use of medications to lyse thrombus in the arterial or venous systems; streptokinase or urokinase are capable of directly or indirectly converting plasminogen to plasmin, which is the active lytic enzyme. Thrombus contains plasminogen, and activation of thrombus-bound plasminogen is the best method of producing thrombolysis.

Recently, tissue plasminogen activator (t-PA) has also been used. This naturally occurring enzyme is present in human tissues in proportion to their vascularity, and can now be produced using recombinant DNA techniques. Since t-PA has a high affinity for activation of thrombus-bound fibrin, relatively selective action can be obtained with few systemic effects.

Thrombolytic agents may be administered systemically (intravenous infusion), or directly into the occluded vessel via an angiographic catheter. Infusion times required to achieve clot dissolution average about 12–36 hours with streptokinase, and 6–18 hours with urokinase, when delivered intra-arterially. Complications include bleeding at the access site, gastrointestinal or cerebral haemorrhage, and allergic reactions to streptokinase.

Regional thrombolytic therapy may be administered percutaneously, using catheter techniques. Regional arterial infusion of low doses of lytic medication into or close to the thrombus is applied in the treatment of acute arterial thrombosis, recent bypass graft occlusion (autogenous or prosthetic), and in the management of thrombotic complications of other intra-arterial interventions).

Where arterial thrombosis occurs at the site of atherosclerotic stenosis, thrombolytic therapy may be used to clear thrombus from the vessel, thus localizing the stenosis and allowing immediate treatment by percutaneous transluminal angioplasty.

Case study 1: Regional thrombolytic infusion of an occluded femoropopliteal bypass graft

This patient presented with a 36 hour history of ischaemia of the right leg which had occurred suddenly two years following placement of a femoropopliteal bypass graft. The femoral pulse was diminished, and the popliteal and distal pulses were absent (Fig. 8.13).

The technique of regional intra-arterial thrombolytic infusion in a clinical case is shown in Fig. 8.14.

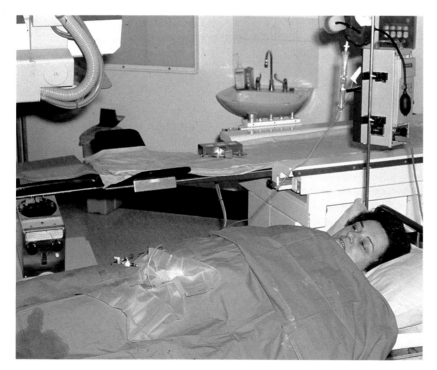

Fig. 8.14 Technique of regional intra-arterial thrombolytic infusion demonstrated in a clinical case. An angiographic catheter has been introduced retrogradely into the left common femoral artery, and fed across the right femoral system for lysis of thrombus within the arteries of the right leg. Patients may be kept in the angiographic suite for several hours to allow progress films to be taken, and are then transferred to an area where close monitoring is available for follow up between angiograms.

Case study 2: Regional thrombolytic infusion with adjunctive balloon angioplasty

This patient presented with relative ischaemia of the leg, 15 months following placement of a femoropopliteal bypass graft (Fig. 8.15).

Case study 3: Regional thrombolytic therapy with adjunctive percutaneous angioplasty

This patient presented with a 24 hour history of ischaemia of the left leg. The initial angiogram demonstrated occlusion of the superficial femoral and popliteal arteries. The sudden onset of symptoms suggested thrombotic occlusion, and a regional infusion of thrombolytic therapy was commenced (Fig. 8.16).

Complications of thrombolytic therapy

Complications of thrombolytic therapy include allergic reactions to streptokinase (urokinase and t-PA are non-allergenic), localized bleeding and bruising, systemic fibrinolysis causing diffuse haemorrhage, gastrointestinal haemorrhage or cerebral bleeding, and embolization of a dislodged clot to distal arteries. Rethrombosis of arteries which have been opened by thrombolytic therapy also occurs frequently (Figs 8.17 and 8.18).

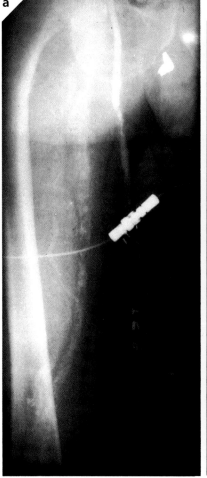
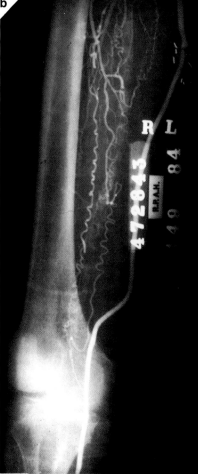

Fig. 8.15 Regional thrombolytic infusion with adjunctive balloon angioplasty. (a) The initial angiogram shows some filling of the proximal portion of the graft which tapers rapidly, with filling defects suggestive of recent thrombosis. **(b)** After 24 hours of thrombolytic medication via a direct intra-arterial catheter, the total length of graft and runoff into the popliteal artery has been re-established. A stenotic region within the graft has been demonstrated, close to the midpoint of the graft where the staples are present on the film. This region of graft stenosis was corrected by percutaneous balloon angioplasty, to protect against rethrombosis.

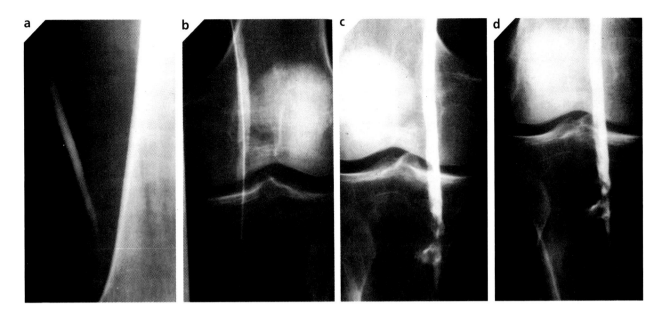

Fig. 8.16 Regional thrombolytic therapy with adjunctive percutaneous angioplasty. (a) The initial film shows results after six hours of therapy, with recanalization of the superficial femoral artery. **(b)** The angiographic infusion catheter is introduced further down into the popliteal system, with recanalization of the proximal popliteal system. **(c)** Recanalization of the entire popliteal artery is seen, with a distal atherosclerotic stenosis and a small region of extravasation caused by the guidewire. **(d)** The final film shows some filling of the tibial artery distal to the stenosis; this stenotic region was considered to be the cause of acute thrombosis, and was treated by immediate percutaneous balloon angioplasty with a satisfactory outcome.

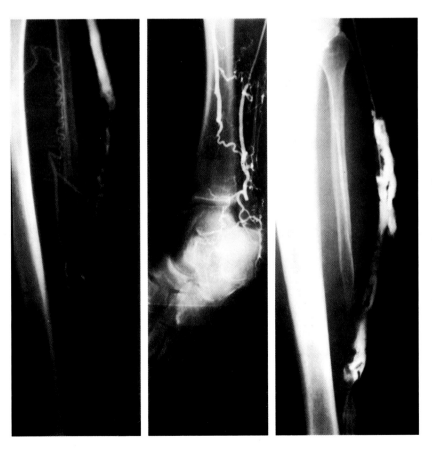

Fig. 8.17 Occlusion of a bypass graft to the anterior tibial artery, treated by regional infusion of thrombolytic therapy. Initially, the recanalization process appeared satisfactory, with refilling of the graft and tibial arteries (centre). However, rethrombosis occurred with considerable build up of thrombotic material within the graft and at athe anastomotic region (right). Partial recanalization, leaving regions of undissolved thrombus within the graft and runoff vessels, is frequently encountered and may be resolved with long term infusion of the lytic agent over 24–48 hours. Alternatively, infusion may be abandoned and surgical measures undertaken.

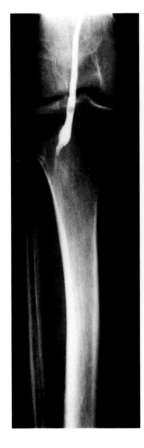 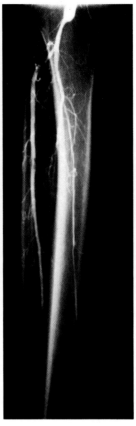 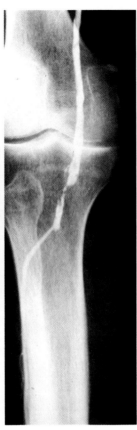

Fig. 8.18 Initially successful thrombolytic therapy, complicated by reocclusion. In this patient, a femoropopliteal bypass graft was reopened with thrombolytic therapy (left and centre). There was evidence of some minor residual thrombus within the distal graft. However, after 12 hours of infusion the clinical condition again deteriorated, and the angiogram revealed occlusion of segments of the bypass and anastomotic region. Simultaneous infusion of heparin is often recommended to prevent occurrence of rethrombosis, but is associated with an increase of bleeding complications.

References

Clagett, G.P., Genton, E., Salzmon, E. (1989) Antithrombotic therapy in peripheral vascular disease. *Chest*, **95**, 1285–395.

Haber, E., Quertermous, T., Matsueda, G.R. and Runge, M.S. (1989) Innovative Approaches to plasminogen activator therapy. *Science*, **243**, 51–6.

Lu, D., Bowman, R.L., Leon, M.B. (1989) Catalytic thermal angioplasty: Catheter design, operating characteristics and preliminary animal results, in *Endovascular Surgery* (eds W.S. Moore and S.S. Ahn). WB Saunders Inc., Philadelphia, PA, pp. 419–28.

Montarjami, A. (1989) Thrombolytic therapy in arterial occlusion and graft thrombosis. *Seminars Vasc. Surg.*, **2**, 155–78.

Siegel, R.J. Fishbein, M.C., Forrester, J. *et al.* (1988) Ultrasonic plaque ablation: A new method for recanalization of partially or totally occluded arteries. *Circulation*, **78**, 1443–8.

Slager, C.J., Essed, C. E., Schuurbiers. J.C.H. *et al.* (1985) Vaporization of atherosclerotic plaques by spark erosion. *J. Am. Coll. Cardiol.*, **5**, 1382–6.

White, G.H., White, R.A., Coleman, P.D., Kopchok, G.E. and Wilson, S.E. (1990) Endoscopic intraluminal surgery removes intraluminal flaps, dissections, and thrombus. *J. Vasc. Surg.*, **11**, 280–8.

White, R.A. and White, W.S. (1989) Alternative laser and thermal angioplasty devices in Lasers, in *Cardiovascular Disease: Clinical Applications, Alternative Angioplasty Devices and Guidance Methods*. Year Book Medical Publishers, Inc., Chicago, Illinois, pp. 141–7.

9 Angioscopy

Angioscopy is a relatively new technique, involving the use of medical endoscopy within the vessels of the vascular system, including intraoperative and percutaneous inspection of the peripheral vascular system and coronary arteries.

The angioscopic techniques and instrumentation have developed rapidly over the last five years, so that angioscopy is now being used more frequently as a diagnostic and therapeutic adjunct for intraoperative peripheral vascular procedures and, more recently, for percutaneous angioplasty. The applications of angioscopy are described in Table 9.1.

EQUIPMENT

Angioscopy is performed with very delicate fibreoptic instruments, which are adapted via a camera attachment for image display on a television screen (Figs 9.1 and 9.2).

Adjunctive components

Adjunctive components consist of high power 300 W light source, television monitor for projection of a 200-fold magnified image, and a video recorder. An intravenous fluid bag is pressurized and connected to a central lumen within the angioscope, for irrigation of the vessel under inspection. Figs 9.3–9.33 demonstrate the different types of angioscopes, ancillary equipment, and methods to achieve visualization during various types of procedures.

Table 9.1 Applications of Angioscopy	
Diagnosis	**Monitoring Vascular Therapies**
Assessment of angiographic findings	Thromboembolectomy and venous thrombectomy
Differentiation of thrombus from atherosclerotic occlusion	Division of venous valves (in situ bypass)
Identification of aortic and arterial dissections	Laser angioplasty, rotational atherectomy and transluminal balloon angioplasty
Intraoperative evaluation of vascular reconstruction	Infusion of thrombolytic agents, vasodilators
Determination of extent of intimal injury due to trauma	Endarterectomy and carotid endarterectomy
Identification of site of venous valves and major tributaries during in situ bypass	
Assessment of coronary artery disease	
Diagnosis of pulmonary embolism	

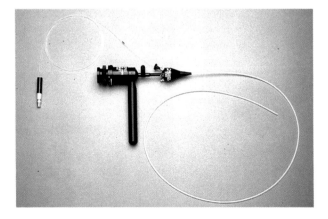

Fig. 9.1 Prototype angioscope. This illustrates the features necessary for endoscopy within the vascular system. The angioscope catheter is narrow. Its size typically ranges between 2–3 mm for intraoperative use in the peripheral vessels, and between 0.5–1.7 mm for use in coronary arteries. The fibreoptic catheter is extremely flexible and has multiple channels for image bundle, light source fibre and fluid irrigation. The model shown here has a handheld eyepiece; the preferred technique is to adapt this eyepiece to a video camera. (Courtesy of Trimedyne Inc., Tustin, CA, USA.)

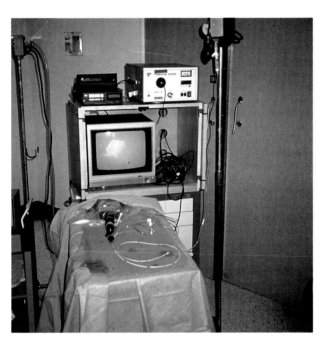

Fig. 9.2 Equipment for intraoperative angioscopy within the femoral and popliteal system. The vascular endoscopy system includes the angioscopy catheter, camera adaptor and video camera (displayed on the sterile field). If the video camera is not sterilizable, it must be put in a sterile plastic bag before taking it into the operative field.

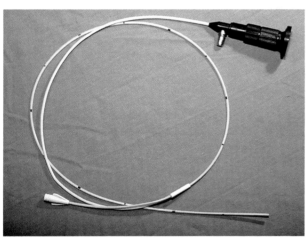

Fig. 9.3 Angioscope catheter for peripheral vessels. Its diameter is 2.3 mm. The eyepiece is attached to the video camera, and an infusion line may be connected to the internal channel of the angioscope.

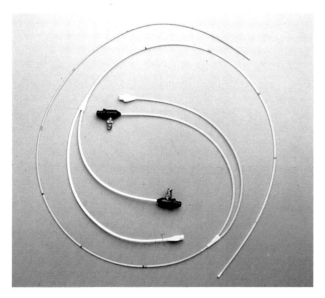

Fig. 9.4 Recently developed, disposable optical catheters. The two catheters shown here are 2.3 mm and 3 mm in diameter, designed to be snap-locked into the light source and camera. These instruments are inexpensive, which means that resterilization is not required. (Courtesy of Baxter Corporation, Santa Ana, CA, USA.)

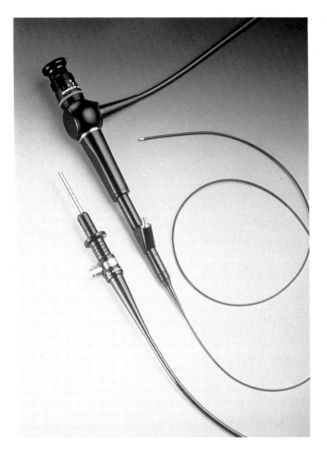

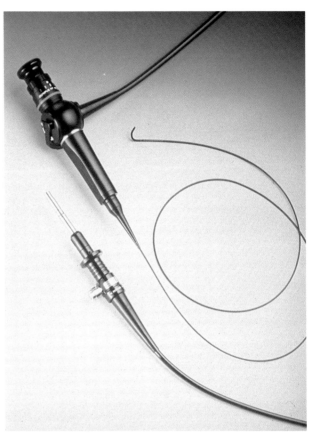

Fig. 9.5 Olympus 2.8 mm angiofibroscope. The light cable is attached to a high intensity light source, because of the small size of the optic fibres. This incorportes a fluid infusion channel and is suitable for use in the iliac, femoral and popliteal arteries. (Courtesy of Olympus Corporation, Lake Success, NY, USA.)

Fig. 9.6 Olympus angioscope with a steerable tip. This endoscope catheter is 2.2 mm in diameter. Because of the size of the internal cables required for deflecting the tip, the fluid infusion channel is omitted from this angioscope; therefore, fluid infusion must be performed via coaxial or adjunctive cannulae. The steerable tip allows more thorough examination of the internal surfaces of the vessel, as well as guided manipulation. (Courtesy of Olympus Corporation, Lake Success, NY, USA.)

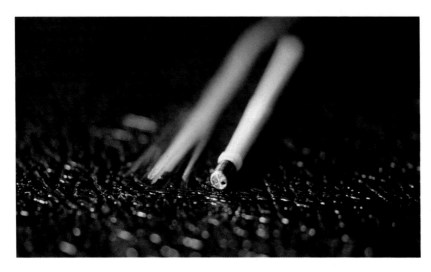

Fig. 9.7 Distal tip of multichannel angioscope. The multiple channels are seen, with the open channel used for fluid irrigation. Most angioscopes have a coherent image bundle consisting of 3000–8000 individual glass or quartz fibres (fibre bundles illustrated on the left), used to bring the image from the distal objective lens to the video equipment. These fibres are quite flexible but likely to break with mistreatment, causing deterioration of the angioscope image.

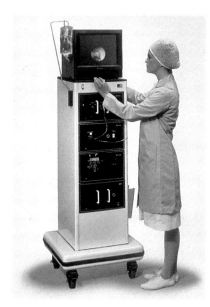

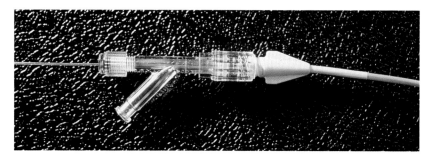

Fig. 9.9 Proximal end of an angioscope. A Y-piece attachment allows passage of various microinstruments, including guidewires and laser fibres, through the internal channel of the angioscope. Fluid irrigation is connected to the other arm of the Y.

Fig. 9.8 Angioscopy system. Manufacturers are now producing fully integrated systems which are more convenient and quicker to set up. The light source, video camera, video recorder and controls are included within a modular box which can be taken into the operating room when required. (Courtesy of Vascucare, Orangeburg, NY, USA.)

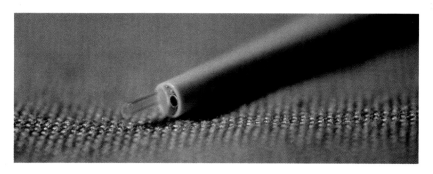

Fig. 9.10 Distal tip of angioscope. A 600 μ laser fibre is seen protruding from the distal end of the working channel of a 2.3 mm diameter angioscope.

Laser angioplasty under direct vision is possible with such a system, but it has not been found practical in patients with widespread atherosclerosis.

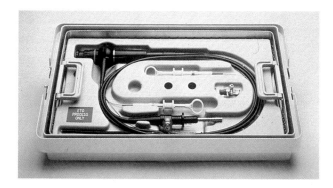

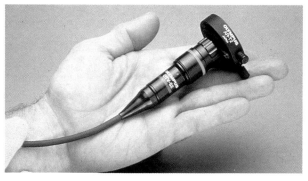

Fig. 9.11 Storage and sterilization tray for angioscope equipment. Angioscopes must be sterilized in ethylene oxide; the process takes between 12–24 hours. In this case, the angioscope is treated with ethylene oxide gas for eight hours at cold temperatures (approximately –130° F), and then allowed to air-dry for a further 6–12 hours so that gas diffuses out of the tubing of the catheter. The casing protects the angioscope from mishandling or damage during the sterilization process, thus preserving the fine optic fibres.

Fig. 9.12 Endoscopic video adaptor. This connects to the head of the angioscope, for transmission of the image to a television screen. This indirect video endoscopy allows preservation of a sterile field. All members of the surgical team are able to observe the magnified image of the video monitor.

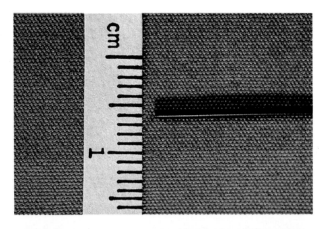

Fig. 9.13 Ultrafine angioscope, of 0.8 mm diameter. This may be used in conjunction with a delivery catheter, to provide irrigation. Such angioscopes of less than 1 mm diameter have been developed for coronary application and use in the smaller peripheral vessels, especially vein grafts and tibial arteries. (Courtesy of Baxter Corporation, Santa Ana, CA, USA.)

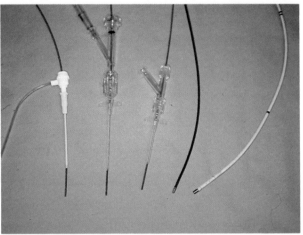

Fig. 9.14 Angioscopes of various sizes and designs. Left: Microfine instruments, between 0.5–1 mm in diameter, with various access cannulae suitable for intraoperative coronary bypass, or for use within the small vessels of the leg. Right: Multichannel angioscope of 2.8 mm diameter, incorporating an internal fluid channel. Second from right: Angioscope of 1.7 mm diameter; it has the same optical bundle as the multichannel angioscope, but no channel for irrigation. It is important that an appropriate design and diameter of angioscope is selected for the various applications, i.e. the multichannel design for intraoperative use, and smaller angioscopes for percutaneous use, with irrigation through a delivery sheath.

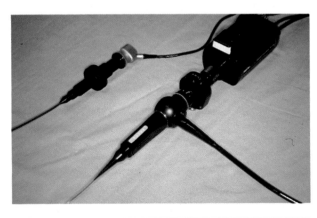

Fig. 9.15 Range of video cameras. Left: Compact medical video camera head, which can be sterilized in ethylene oxide between uses and brought into the sterile field. Right: A larger, non-sterilizable video camera, which must be put in a plastic bag before it is brought into the sterile field. Both types of camera provide good images.

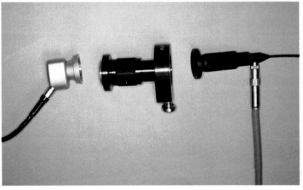

Fig. 9.16 Video adaptor for coupling the angioscope catheter to a video camera. The adaptor includes lenses for magnification and focusing of the endoscopic image.

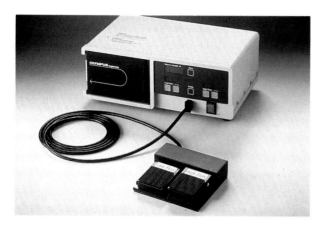

Fig. 9.17 Foot-controlled, fluid irrigation pump.
This provides a maintenance flow of fluid with pressure to one foot pedal, and a flush bolus at a high rate of flow with compression of the second foot pedal. The rates of flow for maintenance and bolus may be set on the control console. Such irrigation systems allow more precise control of the flow of fluid in the patient, and provide a mechanism of high flow rates where blood is occluding the view. (Courtesy of Olympus Corporation, Lake Success, NY, USA.)

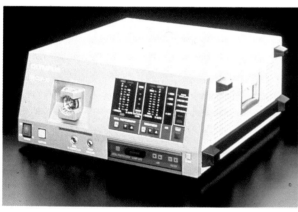

Fig. 9.18 A 300 W light source, used for angioscopy. Many light sources used for medical procedures have power settings of 100–150 W; this power range may not be sufficient for angioscopy, because of the very fine fibres used. Increased light intensity is often required deep within the vascular system.

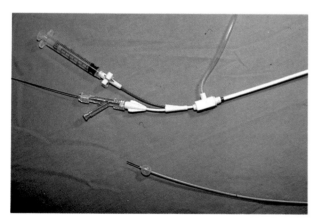

Fig. 9.19 Equipment for percutaneous angioplasty. This illustrates a percutaneous delivery sheath with irrigation side arm, through which a blue 8F angioscope delivery catheter has been introduced. The delivery catheter has an inflatable balloon near its distal tip which is used to occlude the vessel proximal to the site of inspection. The ultrafine angioscope is fed through an internal lumen in the delivery catheter. If there is excessive blood flow in the region, external compression of the artery may be used as an adjunct to control of flow.

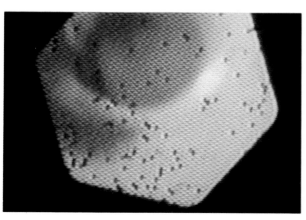

Fig. 9.20 Black spots on angioscope image.
Angioscope catheters are very fragile instruments, because of the glass fibreoptics. If individual fibres break, black spots are produced on the images until the image field is completely covered with them, with deterioration of the optical result. Severe twisting and bending of the angioscope catheter must be avoided, particularly during storage, cleaning and sterilization.

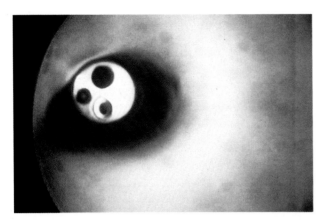

Fig. 9.21 Angioscope catheter tip positioned inside an artery. There is potential for intimal trauma caused by the catheter. However, when the catheter is considerably smaller than the vessel, contact is only over a small part of the tip which is typically smooth to avoid lifting intimal flaps from the vessel wall. The multiple channels of the angioscope catheter are seen.

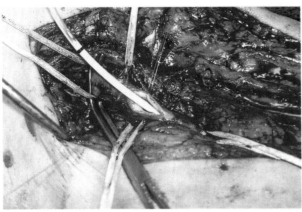

Fig. 9.22 Introduction of angioscope in a peripheral vascular procedure. The inflow of blood has been controlled by clamping the common femoral artery (left of the field), and by placing a loop around the profunda femoris artery (bottom of the field). The angioscope is directed down the superficial femoral artery; there is little backflow of blood, due to distal occlusion of that vessel. The incision made into the artery is that for a bypass operation, and is not changed for the angioscopic procedure.

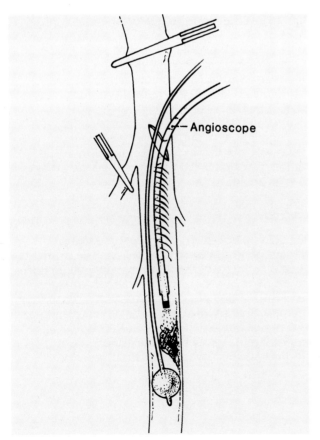

Fig. 9.23 Angioscopy of the superficial femoral artery in a thrombectomy procedure. Diagrammatic representation, showing the clamps on the common and deep femoral arteries, and the angioscope in place. A Fogarty thrombectomy balloon (see page 114) is placed beside the angioscope, and the procedure is directly monitored. (From White and White, 1987, with permission.)

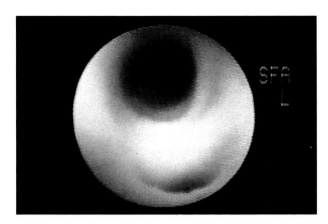

Fig. 9.24 Typical angioscopic appearance of the interior of a normal femoral artery. The artery walls appear white or grey, and show no compromise of the arterial lumen. The opening of a branch vessel is seen near the bottom of the image. Blood has been washed distally, by flow of normal saline through the fluid channel of the angioscope.

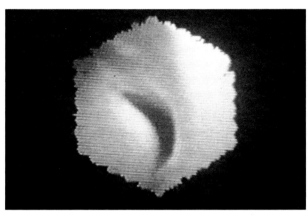

Fig. 9.25 Angioscopic appearance of smooth atheroma of the superficial femoral artery, causing a significant stenosis. The plaque is not showing features of calcification, haemorrhage or ulceration.

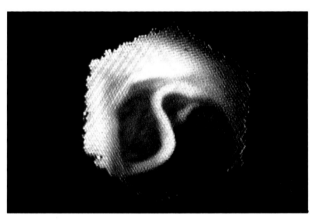

Fig. 9.26 Angioscopic appearance of an intimal flap within the femoral artery. The flap has been complicated by a clot having formed between the flap and vessel wall.

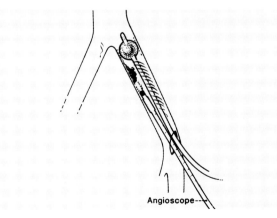

Fig. 9.27 Angioscopy of the iliac artery, via a femoral approach. Diagrammatic representation; for upstream visualization, control of blood inflow must be achieved with a balloon catheter, as shown here. This is quite easily achieved in prosthetic grafts where there is no collateral flow. However, upstream visualization is more difficult in the native arterial system, because of the frequent occurrence of good collateral flow coming in through the lumbar branches of the internal iliac artery. (From White and White, 1987, with permission.)

Angioscope

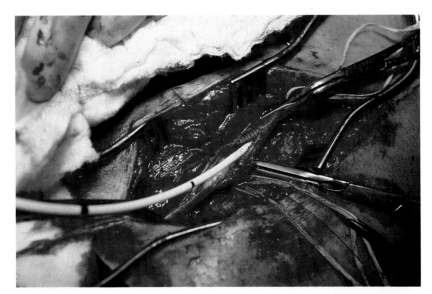

Fig. 9.28 Angioscope introduced, via a retrograde approach, into the occluded limb of an aortobifemoral bypass. In this case, the thrombotic occlusion of the graft prevents blood flow until the thrombus has been removed. After removal, an additional balloon to occlude inflow of blood from the aorta must be introduced to enable further visualization.

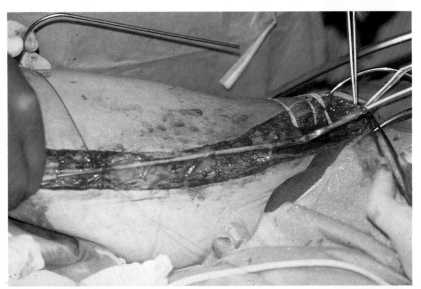

Fig. 9.29 Angioscopic visualization during venous valve ablation for in situ bypass. A retrograde valvulotome is being introduced through a side branch of the exposed saphenous vein, while the angioscope is inserted through the proximal part of the saphenous vein at the groin. Instrumentation of the interior of the vessel may then be observed with an endoscope. As each valve is divided, the angioscope is inserted further down the vein to continue the monitoring procedure.

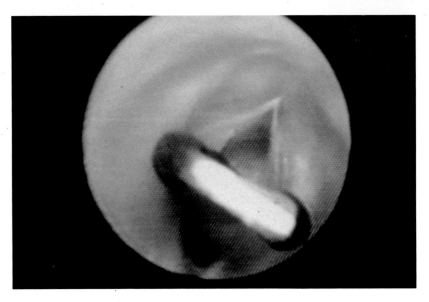

Fig. 9.30 Angioscopic appearance of the valvulotome within the saphenous vein. The head of the valvulotome is positioned over the valve cusp; trauma to the vein may be avoided by accurate monitoring of the procedure.

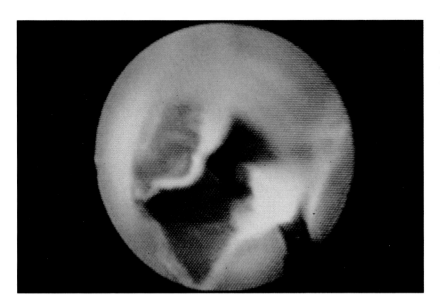

Fig. 9.31 Division of the valve cusp after a single pass with the valvulotome. The cusp is typically torn and shredded, and flow of fluid through the valve region shows it to be incompetent.

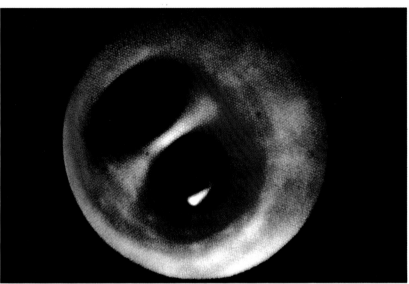

Fig. 9.32 Angioscopic appearance of a side branch of a tributary of the saphenous vein, with the valvulotome in the main channel.

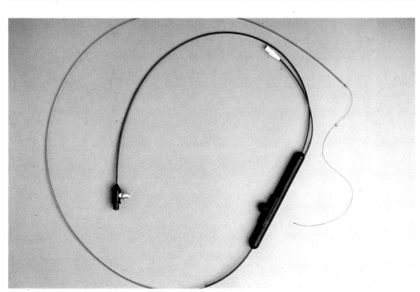

Fig. 9.33 Angioscopic valvulotomy instrument. This Fogarty-Chin device incorporates a cutting blade mechanism inside the angioscope catheter. When the angioscope is advanced to the site of the valve, the prongs of the cutting blade can be advanced to achieve valve division. Direction of the device is aided by a silk suture attached to the leading edge of the valvulotome.

Percutaneous angioscopy

Percutaneous angioscopy (Figs 9.34–9.37) is more difficult than intraoperative use, as the inflow of blood is not well controlled and irriga- tion of the vessel becomes more difficult. External compression of the femoral artery or distal arter- ies may be a useful adjunct to controlling blood flow.

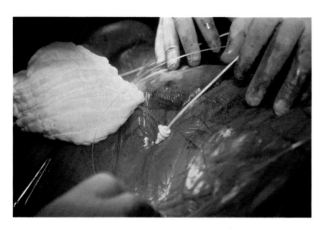

Fig. 9.34 Percutaneous introduction of angioscope. An 8F introducer sheath is inserted into the common femoral artery and directed down the leg. The side arm of the introducer sheath can be used for infusion of fluid, and the angioscope is passed through a haemostatic valve mechanism which prevents bleeding.

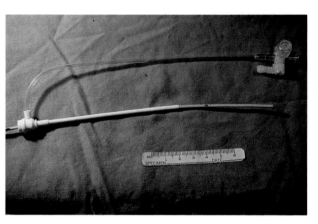

Fig. 9.35 Passage of a multichannel angioscope through an 8F introducing catheter. The side arm has a three-way switch to allow infusion of saline or contrast medium.

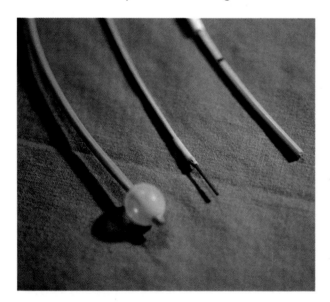

Fig. 9.36 Delivery catheters. Various types are available, allowing atraumatic passage of smaller angioscopes to a more distal site. Here, 6F and 8F delivery catheters with a distal occlusion balloon are shown beside a multichannel 2.3 angioscope (right). (Courtesy of Baxter Corporation, Santa Ana, CA, USA.)

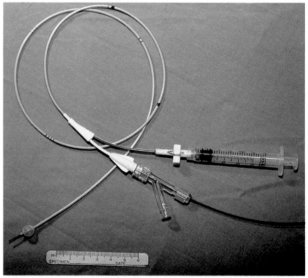

Fig. 9.37 Percutaneous angioscope catheter in detail. The occlusion balloon has been inflated, and the angioscope is seen protruding from the tip of the delivery catheter.

DIAGNOSTIC ANGIOSCOPY

Angioscopy may be used to determine whether a defect seen on arteriography is due to thrombus, embolus or atherosclerosis, when the diagnosis is in doubt. This application should be limited to selected patients; at present, it is best restricted to intraoperative confirmation (Figs 9.38–9.40).

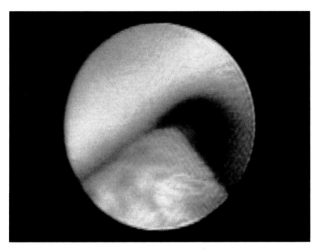

Fig. 9.38 Appearance of a recent, acute thrombus inside a normal vessel.

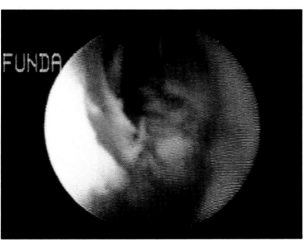

Fig. 9.39 Adherent thrombus overlying a diseased atherosclerotic wall of the profunda femoris artery. This is seen after partial thrombectomy.

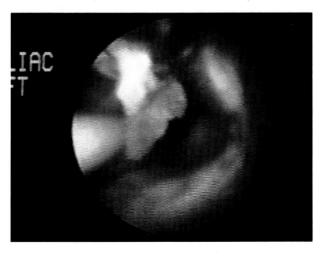

Fig. 9.40 Appearance of a flap of thrombus and intima on the superior wall of the profunda femoris artery. Flaps of tissue or thrombus such as this are frequently missed on the arteriogram, but can be easily illustrated by angioscopy.

References

Angioscopy: Vascular and Coronary Applications (1989) (eds G.H. White and R.A. White), Year Book Medical Publishers, Inc, Chicago, IL.

White, G.H., White, R.A., Kopchok, G.E. *et al.* (1987) Intraoperative video angioscopy compared with angiography during peripheral vascular operations, *J. Vasc. Surg.*, **8**, 488–95.

10 Angioscopic Endovascular Surgical Techniques

ANGIOSCOPIC THROMBOEMBOLECTOMY

The procedure of embolectomy or thrombectomy of occluded peripheral vessels is conventionally performed as a semiclosed procedure, utilizing balloon catheters to extract thrombotic material from the involved artery. As this procedure is performed blindly within a closed vessel, it can lead to inadequate recanalization, inadequate removal of thrombus, or undetected complications of the balloon extraction process.

Angioscopic monitoring of the thromboembolectomy procedure has been shown to have several advantages over the blind procedure. These are listed in Table 10.1. Applications of angioscopy during operative thromboembolectomy procedures are illustrated in Fig. 10.1–10.9.

Table 10.1 Advantages of Angioscopic Thromboembolectomy	
Accurate localization and determination of aetiology of obstruction	Reduction of angiographic contrast and radiation exposure
Guided positioning of thrombectomy catheters	Selective cannulation of major arterial branches
Visual calibration of balloon inflation	Observation of effects of alternative instruments, devices
Immediate detection of retained thrombus	Faster and more convenient than operative angiography
Immediate, accurate detection of complications	
Assessment of underlying atherosclerotic disease	

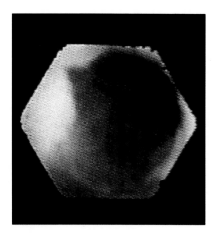

Fig. 10.1 Angioscopic appearance of thrombus within the femoral artery.

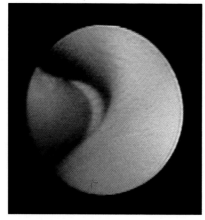

Fig. 10.2 Angioscopic image of the tip of a thrombectomy catheter passing down the femoral artery. The progress of the thrombectomy balloon may be directly observed by passing it alongside the angioscope and removing clot under direct visualization.

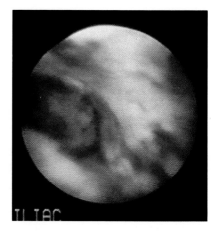

Fig. 10.3 Angioscopic appearance of a large thrombotic occlusion of the iliac artery. This thrombus occurred acutely during a laser angioplasty procedure, and it was detected endoscopically, allowing immediate treatment.

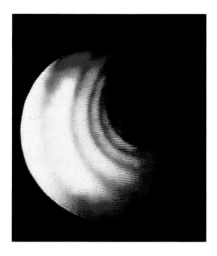

Fig. 10.4 Appearance of thrombus within the lumen of a dacron bypass graft, following several passages of a thrombectomy catheter. One wall of the graft has been cleared very efficiently, while the other wall still shows adherent thrombus.

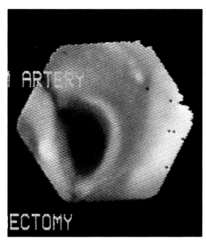

Fig. 10.5 Appearance of superficial femoral artery following thrombectomy. Residual stenosis due to the underlying atherosclerotic process can be seen.

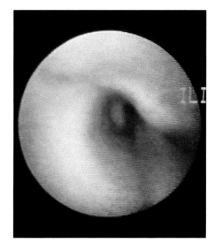

Fig. 10.6 Appearance of stenotic common iliac artery after clearance of thrombus. The reddish tubing of the Fogarty embolectomy balloon catheter is shown; the balloon is inflated proximally to occlude blood flow. The discovered stenosis was treated by intraoperative balloon dilatation.

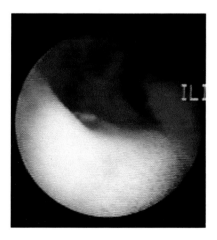

Fig. 10.7 Appearance of the vessel after dilatation of the stenotic lesion, showing widened lumen.

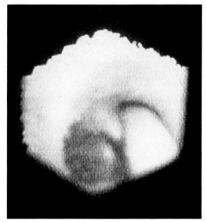

Fig. 10.8 Angioscopy allows guided manipulation of the embolectomy catheter into separate arterial branches below the knee. Passage of the catheter tip into the tibioperioneal trunk is shown, while a large piece of thrombus is seen within the orifice of the anterior tibial artery. The balloon catheter can be guided into the various branches to achieve a more complete removal of thrombus.

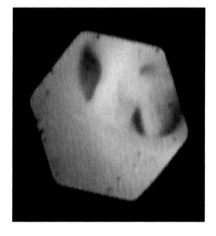

Fig. 10.9 Appearance of a piece of embolic debris within the orifice of the anterior tibial artery. This is of moderate size. The embolectomy balloon preferentially passed down the other branch, but could be introduced into the anterior tibial orifice after a small twist was formed at the distal tip of the catheter. The embolus was then retrieved, with return of the dorsalis pedis pulse.

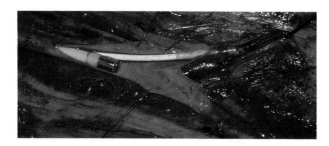

Fig. 10.10 Guided passage of balloon catheters into a side branch in an animal model. The vessel has been opened to show the side of the angioscope catheter placed near the vessel branch; the balloon catheter has been successfully directed into the smaller side branch.

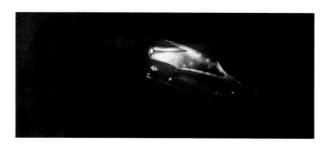

Fig. 10.11 Internal view of the same process, illuminated by the angioscope light source. The position of the angioscope is seen in relation to the catheter, as illustrated in Figs 10.8 and 10.10.

The application of angioscopy during clearance of occlusion in the limb of an aortobifemoral bypass graft is illustrated in Figs 10.12–10.17.

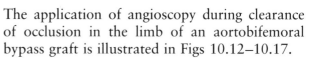

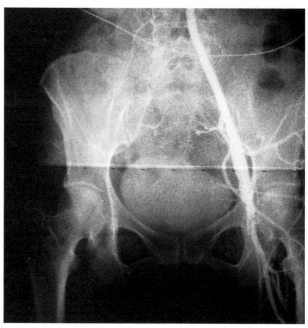

Fig. 10.12 Preoperative angiogram of an ischaemic leg. This patient presented with recent ischaemia of the right leg at an interval of two years after placement of an aortobifemoral bypass graft. The right femoral pulse was absent, and the angiogram confirmed total occlusion of the right limb of the graft.

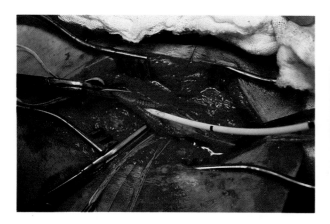

Fig. 10.13 Introduction of the angioscope catheter. Following thrombectomy of the graft limb with a balloon catheter, the angioscope catheter was introduced to inspect the interior of the graft. At this stage, flow of blood through the graft was poor.

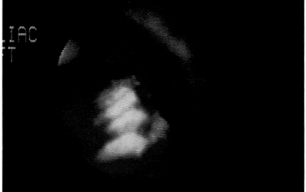

Fig. 10.14 Endoscopic examination of the segment of graft near the femoral anastomosis. This revealed a prominent 'kink' in the posterior wall of the prosthesis, which was due to excessive tension on the graft limb. This was easily corrected by extension of the graft with an additional segment of prosthetic material. Further passage of the balloon catheter cleared more thrombus from the graft wall.

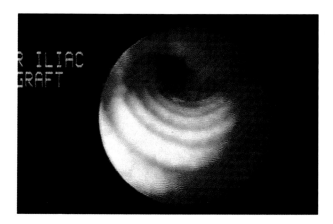

Fig. 10.15 Endoscopic inspection of the proximal segment of the graft. This showed that there was significant thrombus still remaining on the graft wall.

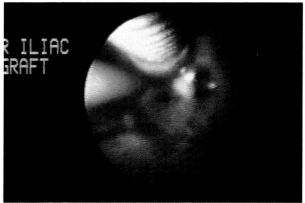

Fig. 10.16 Endoscopic inspection of the bifurcation of the graft. A large plug of thrombotic material remained, which was resistant to removal by the embolectomy balloon. A pair of flexible biopsy forceps were utilized to extract the residual material. The balloon catheter (blue), inflated proximal to the area of manipulation, is illustrated, together with the biopsy forceps (silver) used to retrieve material.

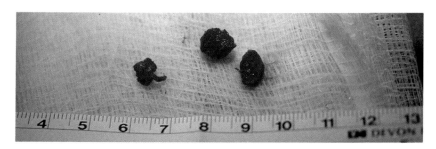

Fig. 10.17 Portions of occlusive material removed from the graft bifurcation. Excellent flow through the graft was established, and the graft limb was salvaged.

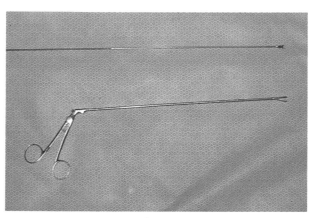

Fig. 10.18 Forceps used in angioscope removal of thrombus and intimal flaps. The rigid biopsy forceps (below) are suitable for larger, straight segments of artery, such as the iliac artery or prosthetic grafts, whereas the flexible bronchial biopsy forceps (above) may be used in the femoral and popliteal arteries. Careful, gentle application is required to avoid trauma to the vessel wall.

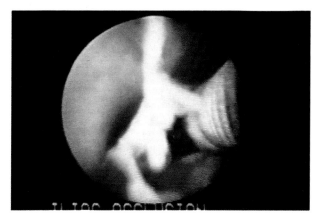

Fig. 10.19 Example of endoscopic removal of a flap of organized thrombus from the wall of the iliac artery. Thrombosis had occurred after insertion of an intra-aortic balloon pump. Much of the thrombus had become adherent to the arterial wall and was difficult to extract with a balloon catheter, but it was successfully retrieved by the biopsy forceps with angioscopic monitoring.

ENDOSCOPIC INTRAVASCULAR SURGERY

With the recent trend towards less invasive techniques of management of medical and surgical disorders, there has been increased emphasis on the use of endoscopic procedures as alternatives to traditional surgical operations. Angioscopy allows direct monitoring of many vascular interventions that were previously performed blindly or by radiological monitoring alone.

The concept of endoscopic intravascular surgery has been developed. In its simplest form, endoscopic intravascular surgery involves removal of residual thrombus or intimal flaps from the vessel wall using forceps of various types, with angioscopic monitoring (Figs 10.20 and 10.21). More complex interventions and manipulation within the vascular system are being developed and controlled by angioscopy.

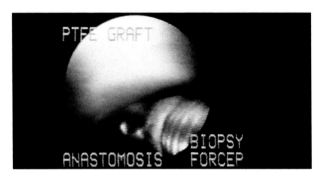

Fig. 10.20 Biopsy forceps grasping material from the anastomotic region of a PTFE graft anastomosed to the popliteal artery. Similar manipulations have been used in an attempt to remove neointimal hyperplasia from the anastomotic region of occluded prosthetic grafts, particularly at the distal anastomosis.

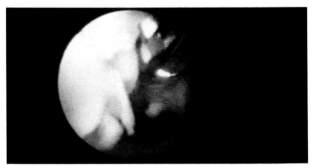

Fig. 10.21 Same procedure of removal of neointimal hyperplasia and residual thrombus from the anastomotic region. The head of the biopsy forceps is seen above material grasped from the left side of the anastomotic wall.

ENDOSCOPIC REMOVAL OF TRAUMATIC INTIMAL FLAP

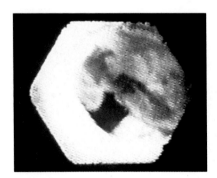

Fig. 10.22 Appearance of the popliteal artery after passage of a balloon catheter introduced from the femoral approach. Some thrombus has been removed from this vessel, but a lot of it is still adherent to the vessel wall. Repeat balloon thrombectomy was performed.

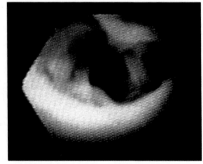

Fig. 10.23 Appearance of the same vessel after repeat balloon thrombectomy procedure. This shows residual thrombus and a flap of intima which had been caused by the initial trauma.

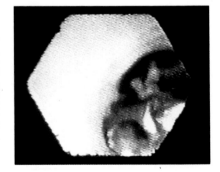

Fig. 10.24 Biopsy forceps being used to grasp the intimal flap for removal via the intravascular route.

CASE STUDIES

Endoscopic removal of thrombus and intimal flaps after vascular trauma

Biopsy forceps and other instruments are used for removing residual thrombus and intimal flaps caused by penetrating or blunt vascular trauma. A series of endoscopic views (Figs 10.22–10.27) shows manipulations undertaken within the popliteal artery in a young male who had suffered thrombotic occlusion of that artery, associated with posterior dislocation of the knee which occurred during a motorcycle accident.

Removal of intimal flap after brachial artery gunshot injury

This patient suffered a shotgun injury to the brachial artery. A traumatized section of artery was resected and replaced with end-to-end reversed vein graft, but inspection of the proximal artery through the vein graft revealed unsuspected intimal flap within the artery. This was treated by removal with forceps under angioscopic visualization (Figs 10.28–10.30).

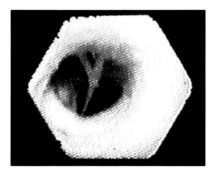

Fig. 10.25 Appearance following removal of the initial segment of intimal flap. A small portion of residual flap is revealed.

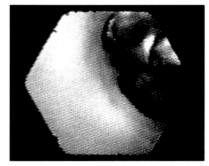

Fig. 10.26 Repeat passage of biopsy forceps. This results in the removal of the entire plane of the intimal flap and successful recanalization of the vessel.

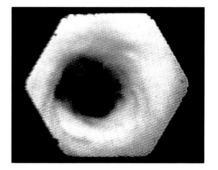

Fig. 10.27 Final appearance of the popliteal artery after removal of thrombus and intimal flap. Successful patency was maintained following the procedure.

Removal of intimal flap from brachial artery

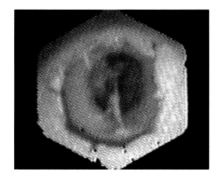

Fig. 10.28 Endoscopic view of the proximal brachial artery. Visualization through the anastomosis upstream. Intimal flap and residual debris are seen; externally, the artery had appeared normal.

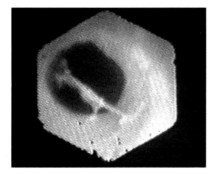

Fig. 10.29 Some of the debris was removed with flexible biopsy forceps, leaving a minor intimal flap.

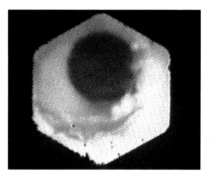

Fig. 10.30 Appearance of the anastomotic region and proximal artery after removal of most of the debris and intimal flaps. Satisfactory function of the bypass graft was achieved.

Removal of intravascular foreign body with endoscopic monitoring

Angioscopy can be used for monitoring the removal of intravascular foreign bodies with various grasping forceps or other instruments. In this case, a shotgun pellet embolus was removed from the tibial artery (Figs 10.31 and 10.32).

ANGIOSCOPY AS AN ADJUNCT TO LASER ANGIOPLASTY

Angioscopy has potential applications for intravascular guidance of laser fibres for positioning and aiming of the laser probe. It can also be used for immediate inspection of the vessel lumen following the laser procedure, to assess the adequacy of recanalization and occurrence of complications (Figs 10.33–10.35).

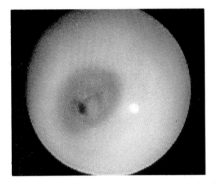

Fig. 10.31   Endoscopic view of pellet embolus in the lumen of the artery, near the orifice of a small branch.

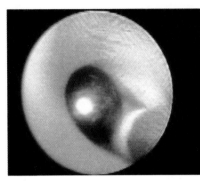

Fig. 10.32   Introduction of an embolectomy balloon catheter. This is inflated just distal to the foreign body, and is retracted gently to avoid trauma to the arterial wall.

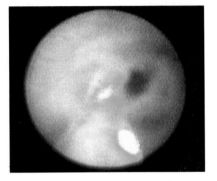

Fig. 10.33   Appearance of a fibreoptic laser probe within a diseased femoral artery. This is during application of Argon laser energy to the region of vascular occlusion. The Argon light causes a characteristic blue/green illumination within the vessel.

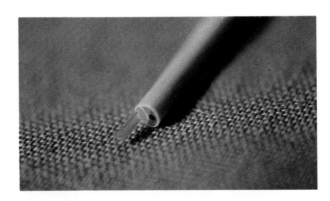

Fig. 10.34   Laser energy via fibreoptics to an atherosclerotic plaque. The laser fibre is fed through the instrumentation channel of the angioscope, allowing direct visual monitoring of the laser ablation procedure. This technique remains investigational; direct application of laser energy was only capable of forming a small channel through the lesion. Furthermore, endoscopic monitoring requires irrigation with clear fluid, which attenuates the laser energy.

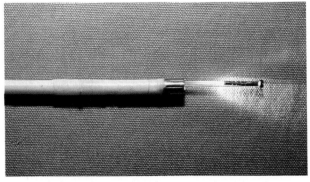

Fig. 10.35   Application of hot tip laser thermal energy with the laser fibre fed through the instrumentation channel of an angioscope. The laser thermal probe is seen projecting forwards from the tip of the angioscope, illuminated by the light source. This technique has been used experimentally; in clinical use, the laser fibre is usually fed alongside the angioscope rather than through its internal channel.

ANGIOSCOPIC APPEARANCES OF LASER RECANALIZATION

The angioscope can be used at various stages during laser recanalization, to monitor progress and adequacy of the procedure (Figs 10.36–10.47). Common features include thermal damage, intimal dissection and fragmentation, mural thrombus and tissue flaps.

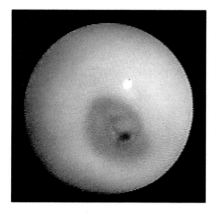

Fig. 10.36 Preoperative appearance of the iliac artery in the region of a 15 cm occlusion. The angioscope has been inserted through the femoral artery; the external iliac artery is relatively normal, leading to a very tight, tapered stenosis and an occlusive lesion of the common iliac artery. The laser probe tends to follow the plane of least resistance, which in this case is the tapered stenosis.

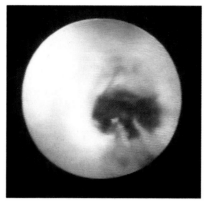

Fig. 10.37 Appearance of the occluded segment of artery following the passage of a 2.5 mm laser thermal probe. A narrow channel has been formed within the occlusion, with some fragmentation and thermal injury to the side walls.

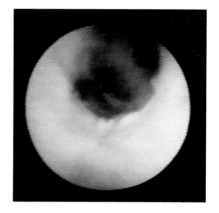

Fig. 10.38 Appearance following adjunctive balloon dilatation. This shows the increased lumen size, achieved without obvious wall dissection or other complications. This patient had an excellent clinical result, with recanalization of the previously occluded segment and return of distal pulses.

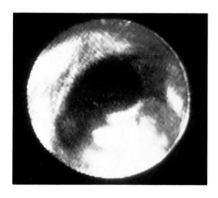

Fig. 10.39 Appearance of a popliteal artery following laser assisted balloon angioplasty. The vessel has been recanalized, but there is significant residual atheroma in the posterior wall, typical wall cracks caused by balloon dilatation, and some associated intramural haemorrhage together with mural thrombus.

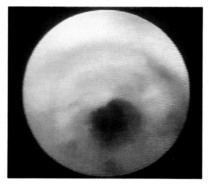

Fig. 10.40 Appearance of a vessel following passage of the laser probe alone. Even with successful passage of the larger 2.5 mm and 3.5 mm probes, the outcome in the lumen is usually inadequate and adjunctive balloon angioplasty is almost always required. This limitation may be dealt with by the introduction of larger probes or multiple array laser fibres.

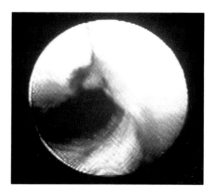

Fig. 10.41 Appearance of a treated, superficial femoral artery. This shows some degree of laser thermal damage to the wall, and mural cracks due to the balloon dilatation.

121

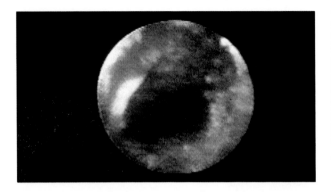

Fig. 10.42   Example of severe thermal damage to the wall of a superficial femoral artery. There is evident charring and coagulation of blood against the wall.

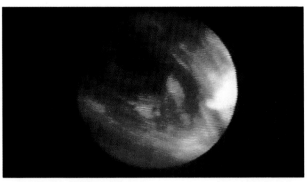

Fig. 10.43   Appearance of an iliac artery after passage of a 3.5 mm laser probe. In this case, the vessel has been recanalized quite successfully, and there is typical fragmentation of the wall lining leaving small flaps within the lumen.

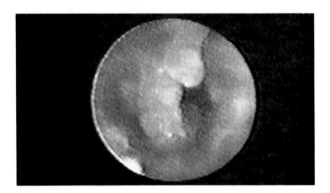

Fig. 10.44   Appearance of acute thrombosis following passage of the laser fibre. In this case, large clumps of thrombotic material are present within the lumen, resulting in acute reocclusion.

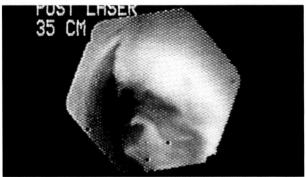

Fig. 10.45   Appearance of a popliteal artery following passage of a 4.2 mm laser probe. The previously occluded vessel has been recanalized; however, the new lumen is very ragged and inadequate for long term patency. The cracks in the atheroma due to passage of the large probe are similar to those caused by balloon dilatation.

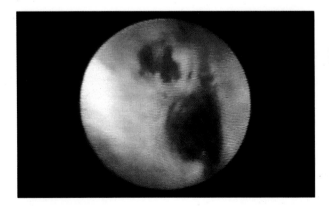

Fig. 10.46   Appearance of a false channel within the wall of the iliac artery. This was caused by passage of the laser probe. The main channel (below) was subsequently dilated with a balloon, giving a satisfactory result.

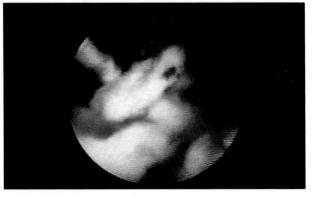

Fig. 10.47   Appearance of debris adherent to the arterial wall following laser assisted balloon angioplasty. It is common for the wall to have such an appearance in the region where the most severe atherosclerotic disease was present.

CORONARY ANGIOSCOPY

Endoscopy of the coronary arteries can be performed as an intraoperative procedure during bypass operation. In selected instances it may be performed percutaneously. The percutaneous technique is quite difficult and demanding, requiring sophisticated delivery catheters and intermittent balloon occlusion of the orifice of the coronary artery.

Intraoperative coronary angioscopy requires special delivery catheters, to enable atraumatic entry of the very fine angioscope catheter into the coronary artery or bypass graft (Figs 10.48–10.50).

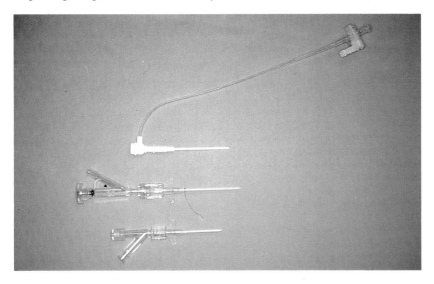

Fig. 10.48 Range of fine intravenous cannulae used for intraoperative coronary angioscopy. The angioscope may be fed through the central lumen of cannulae such as these, so that fluid irrigation may be carried out simultaneously. If used carefully, the soft cannula tip is atraumatic.

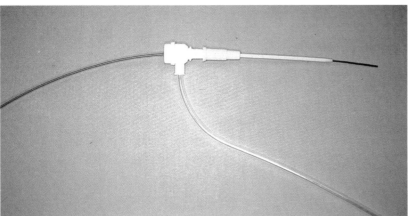

Fig. 10.49 Ultrafine angioscope, less than 1 mm in diameter, fed through the central lumen of the delivery catheter. The delivery catheter incorporates a haemostatic valve and side arm for fluid irrigation.

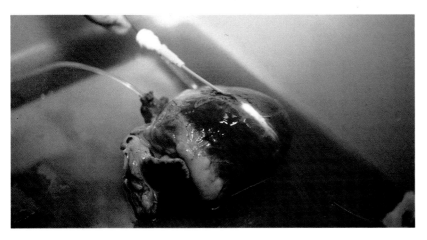

Fig. 10.50 Experimental method of intraoperative angioscopy in an animal model. The delivery cannula has been fed through a surgical arteriotomy into the coronary artery, and is used for introduction of the angioscope further down the vessel. The light from the angioscope is illuminating the interior of the coronary artery.

INTRAOPERATIVE CORONARY ANGIOSCOPY

Applications of this technique are illustrated in Figs 10.51–10.60.

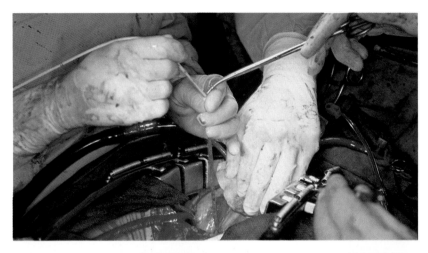

Fig. 10.51 In a coronary artery bypass graft, the angioscope is introduced into the proximal end of a saphenous vein. The distal anastomosis has been made to the coronary artery, and the angioscope is used to inspect the anastomotic region.

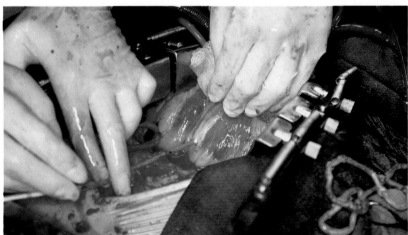

Fig. 10.52 Manipulation of the bypass graft, allowing full examination of the anastomotic region. Here the graft has been reflected downwards, while the heart is being held steady by an assistant.

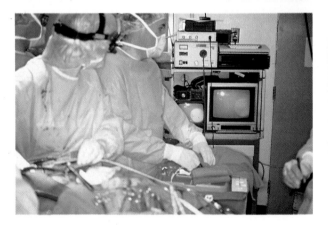

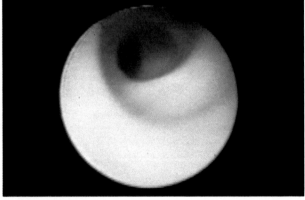

Fig. 10.53 Surgeon watching the video monitor during manipulations. The monitor gives a highly magnified image of the coronary anastomosis. An assistant ensures adequate illumination, and controls the rate of fluid irrigation (using cardioplegia solution).

Fig. 10.54 Endoscopic appearance of a cardiac vein at its site of entry into the coronary sinus, in an animal experiment. The cardiac veins typically demonstrated a spiral, fold-like appearance, with small valves at the entry into the coronary sinus.

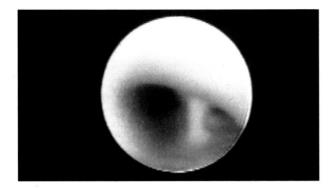

Fig. 10.55 Normal appearance of the distal aspect of the left anterior descending coronary artery, at its point of bifurcation. The walls are non-diseased, and appear white or light blue in colour. Passage of the endoscope to this point must be performed very carefully, so that intimal flaps will not be raised by the tip of the catheter.

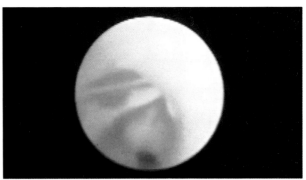

Fig. 10.56 Region of intimal trauma caused by the angioscope tip, in an animal model. If the catheter is forced through a region of vessel tortuosity, it is quite easy to lift a layer of intima causing a traumatic dissection.

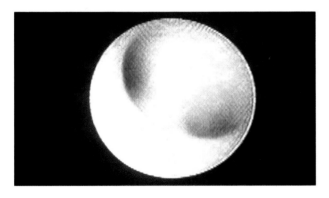

Fig. 10.57 Appearance of the terminal branches of the right coronary artery. Healthy arterial wall is seen.

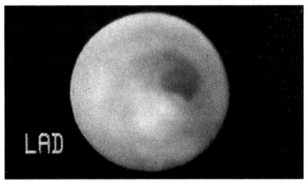

Fig. 10.58 Intraoperative view of mild arterial stenosis. This is associated with atherosclerosis of the left anterior descending coronary artery, distal to the point of proposed bypass.

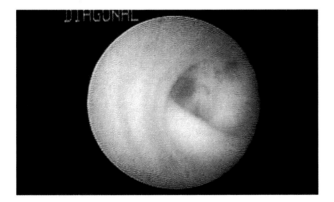

Fig. 10.59 Appearance of the anastomotic region of a vein graft to the diagonal artery. The distal portion of the vein graft (including a valve) is shown, with the suture line evident at the point of anastomosis to the diagonal artery.

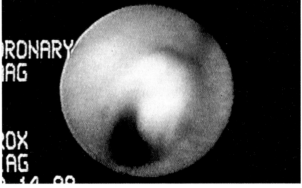

Fig. 10.60 A large, smooth plaque is seen within the wall of the artery, causing approximately 50% stenosis of this vessel. In this case, the angioscope was used to inspect the lesion within a diagonal artery, proximal to the site of anastomosis.

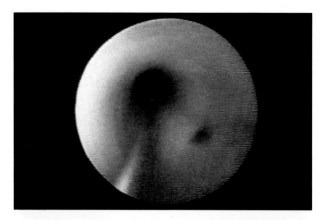

OTHER APPLICATIONS OF ANGIOSCOPY

Fig. 10.61 Endoscopic direction of guidewire insertion. A guidewire has been inserted through the fluid channel of the angioscope, and is seen progressing down the vessel where it may be directed into selected branches with angioscopic control.

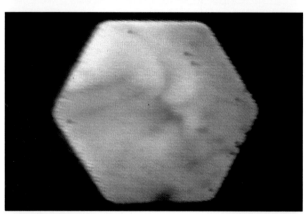

Fig. 10.62 Angioscopic appearance of the anastomosis of a saphenous vein to the popliteal artery. The hood of the graft is seen above the suture line, and the native arterial wall is below with the opening of the side branch at the 5 o'clock position. Inspection of the anastomotic suture line may be used to exclude technical errors such as misplaced sutures, intimal flaps and acute thrombosis.

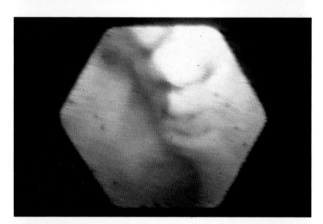

Fig. 10.63 Anastomotic suture line of a prosthetic graft to the popliteal artery. The internal wall of the prosthesis is seen on the right, the suture line in the centre and the wall of the native artery on the left. The sutures are well placed, and no technical defect is detected. In this way, angioscopy can be used to replace other methods of monitoring bypass grafts intraoperatively. However, angioscopy is limited by the amount of runoff artery that can be inspected.

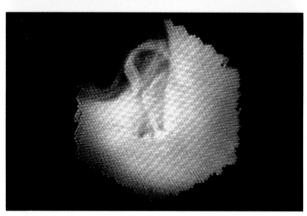

Fig. 10.64 Angioscopic appearance of a small intimal flap. This was caused by instrumentation within the superficial femoral artery. Such small flaps may be the nidus for subsequent thrombosis, and in selected cases they can be removed with endoscopy.

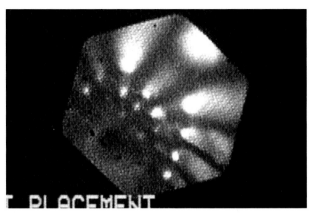

Fig. 10.65 Angioscopic appearance of the interior of a metallic vascular stent. The stent has been placed and expanded over a balloon catheter in a region of vascular stenosis.

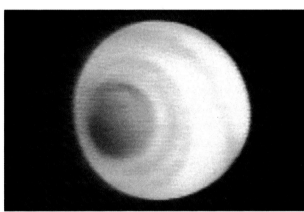

Fig. 10.66 Endoscopic appearance of the interior of a stent. This had been placed in an experimental animal artery three months previously. The spiral metallic struts of this particular stent have been completely covered by endothelium without significant neointimal hyperplasia, and with maintenance of an excellent vessel lumen.

References

Abela, G., Seeger, J.M., Barbieri, E. *et al.* (1986) Laser angioplasty with angioscopic guidance in human, *J. Amer. Coll. Cardiol.*, **8**, 184–92.

Forrester, J.S., Litvack, F. Grundfest, W., *et al.* (1987) A perspective of coronary disease seen through the arteries of living man, *Circulation*, **75**, 505–13.

Grundfest, W.S., Litvack, F., Glick, D., Sogalowirz, J., Treiman, R., Cohen, L., Foren, R., Levin, P., Cossmaru, D., Carroll, R., Spigelman, A., Forrester, J. (1988) Intraoperative decisions based on angioscopy in peripheral vascular surgery, *Circulation*, **78** (Suppl. 1), **1**, 13–17.

Grundfest, W.S., Litvack, F., Sherman, F., Sherman, T. *et al.* (1985) Delineation of peripheral and coronary detail by intraoperative angioscopy, *Ann. Surg.*, **202**, 394–400.

Mehigan, J.T. and DeCampil, W., (1989) Angioscopic control of carotid endarterectomy, in *Endovascular Surgery* (eds W. Moore and S. Ahn), WB Saunders Co., Philadelphia, PA.

Mehigan, J.T. and Olcott, C. (1986) Video angioscopy as an alternative to intraoperative arteriography, *Am. J. Surg.*, **152**, 139–45.

Vollmar, J.F., Storz, L.W. (1974) Vascular endoscopy, *Surg. Clin. North. Am.* **54**, 111–22.

White, R.A. and White, G.H. (1988) Angioscopic monitoring of laser angioplasty, in (eds G.H. White and R.A. White) *Angioscopy: Vascular and Coronary Applications*, Year Book Medical Publishers, Chicago, IL.

White, G.H., White, R.A., Kopchok, G.E. *et al.* (1988) Angioscopic thromboembolectomy: Preliminary experiences with a recent technique, *J. Vasc. Surg.*, **7**, 318–25.

White, G.H., White, R.A., Kopchok, G.E. *et al.* (1990) Endoscopic intravascular surgery removes intraluminal flaps, dissections and thrombus. *J. Vasc. Surg*, **11**, 280–8.

11 Imaging Techniques in Vascular Surgery

Precise guidance of intraluminal angioplasty devices, particularly through high resistance occlusive lesions, is a limiting factor which must be addressed by further development, if improved instruments and clinical results are to be achieved.

Recanalization of distal, small diameter peripheral arteries and coronary lesions requires control with a sensitivity equivalent to the thickness of a vessel wall (approximately 200–300 μm). This degree of precision enables passage of devices through a vessel without causing perforation or false aneurysm formation. Thus, the challenge lies in the application of methods which permit reproducible concentric recanalization of a vessel, while still preserving a relatively uniform thickness of the media and adventitia of the wall.

Spectroscopy and angioscopy have already been addressed as methods of intravascular guidance (see Chapters 5 and 9). Advanced fluoroscopic equipment and ultrasound (both transcutaneous external and intraluminal) are systems which pro-

vide improved and precise intraluminal guidance, and will be addressed in the following discussion.

FLUOROSCOPY

Fluoroscopy is readily available, and is the standard method of quantitating the luminal anatomy of arterial disease. It provides a detailed outline of the location and severity of stenoses and occlusions, and is uniformly applied in the guidance of devices. Fluoroscopy is also used to determine the success of interventional procedures.

Standard angiographic techniques, which often lack good spatial and contrast resolution, may require multiple reinjections to follow progress of the dye. Digital subtraction techniques have increased contrast sensitivity, allowing detection of low levels of iodinated contrast. Many digital units have freeze-frame and roadmapping features which permit superimposition of a subtracted contrast image of a vessel on a live fluoroscopic image (Figs 11.1 and 11.2).

In modern interventional radiology departments, cardiac catheterization laboratories and

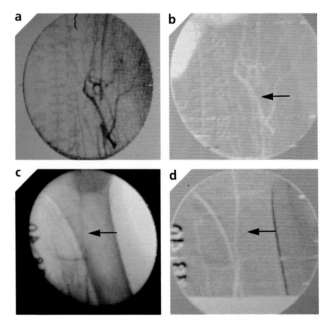

Fig. 11.1 Roadmapping capabilities allow the live fluoroscopic image of a 2.5 mm diameter laser thermal probe to be superimposed on the subtraction contrast outline of the artery being treated. (From White, White and Kopchok, 1989, with permission.)

Fig. 11.2 Display of images stored during the laser angioplasty shown in Fig. 11.1. (a) Arteriogram and (b) image-enhanced roadmap of an occlusion in the superficial femoral artery (arrows). (c) Arteriogram taken immediately after recanalization, showing a small patent lumen (arrow). (d) Subtraction contrast outline of the recanalized segment prior to further treatment to enlarge the lumen.

operating theatres, the quality of equipment available for radiological imaging in surgery varies from conventional C-arm fluoroscopes to sophisticated image-intensifying tubes, high resolution intensifiers, and television monitoring systems. Immediate image replay systems can improve the accuracy of information conveyed, as well as the safety of interventional procedures. Unfortunately, this type of equipment is expensive, and is not available in many surgical departments. An example of a new imaging system which is especially suited for angioplasty procedures in the operating room is shown in Fig. 11.3.

Recent advances in computerized image processing systems enhance the advantages of digital imaging technology to C-arm fluoroscopy, by enabling modular addition of contrast enhancement, image holding and roadmapping during angiographic procedures (Figs 11.4 and 11.5).

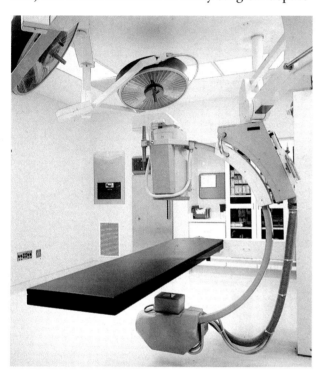

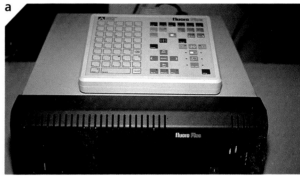

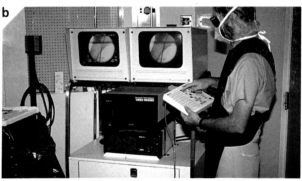

Fig. 11.3 Operating theatre equipped with ceiling-suspended X-ray system and carbon fibre surgical table. The latter provides unobstructed fluoroscopic visualization, and is wall-mounted to enable access over the entire length of the patient. (Courtesy of International Surgical Systems, Phoenix, Arizona, USA.)

Fig. 11.4 Computerized image processing system (a), mounted below fluoroscopy screens (b), enables addition of digital touch pad control to obtain contrast enhancement, image holding and roadmapping to C-arm systems. This system was used to obtain the images displayed in Figs 11.1 and 11.2.

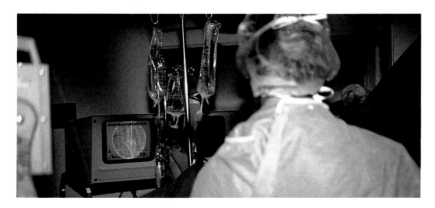

Fig. 11.5 Contrast-enhanced images and roadmaps are easily observed by the physician performing the angioplasty, in the interventional surgery theatre or operating room table.

Limitations of fluoroscopic guidance

Atherosclerotic occlusions of arteries develop with an eccentric positioning inside the vessel lumen, in approximately 70% of both coronary and peripheral lesions (see Chapter 1). Because of the asymmetrical location of the residual lumen, contrast radiology shows significant variability in the estimation of the percentage of luminal stenosis, as it only visualizes the vessel in one dimension (Figs 11.6 and 11.7).

An additional consequence of the eccentric positioning of atherosclerotic lesions is that angiography is unable to determine the transmural component of a lesion (Fig. 11.8).

VASCULAR ULTRASOUND IMAGING
Transcutaneous duplex and colour flow ultrasound

Non-invasive, vascular diagnostic techniques are playing an increasingly important role in the laboratory assessment of the haemodynamic significance of atherosclerotic disease. These techniques involve doppler measurement of pressure indices, analysis of arterial waveforms and emitted sound spectra, as well as ultrasound imaging of the morphology of the vessel wall or atheromatous plaques.

Transcutaneous duplex scanner images have also been evaluated for guidance of angioplasty

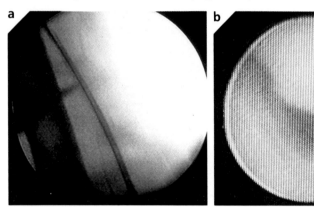

Fig. 11.6 Angiogram of a superficial femoral artery. This is an anteroposterior projection which appears to be normal (**a**). A 0.32″ guidewire is also seen, which was easily passed through the lumen. (**b**) Angioscopic inspection of the vessel lumen reveals a large (approximately 60%) stenosis in the vessel, produced by a lesion on the posterior wall.

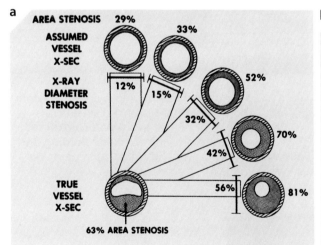

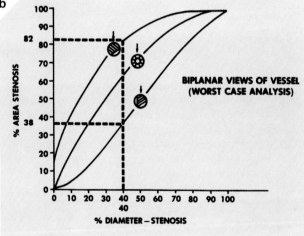

Fig. 11.7 Measurement of areas of stenosis in asymmetrical lesions. (**a**) The assumed or apparent degrees of diameter and area of stenosis are given, when an asymmetrical lesion is visualized through different projections. (**b**) The relationship between the area and diameter of stenosis is shown when the artery is asymmetrically narrowed (top and bottom lines), and when it is symmetrically narrowed (middle line). The arrows indicate the direction of the X-ray beam in the projection showing the greatest degrees of narrowing. If the stenosis is asymmetrical, and if two orthogonal views are assumed, the actual area of stenosis must lie between the upper and lower lines. Only if the stenosis is symmetrical can a precise estimate of the area be obtained. (From Sumner, Russell and Miles, 1983, with permission.)

devices through lesions in the vessel lumen. Computerized, colour-coded duplex ultrasound imaging is proving particularly valuable in detecting and quantifying atherosclerotic disease of the peripheral vascular system (Figs 11.9–11.18). This may be used to select patients who are suitable for less invasive modes of treatment by endovascular surgical techniques. Subsequent progress

of the treated lesions may then be followed by consecutive scans.

Overall, ultrasound devices are the most promising means of permitting a three-dimensional guidance of angioplasty instruments. They also facilitate non-invasive follow up examinations for detecting recurrence of lesions.

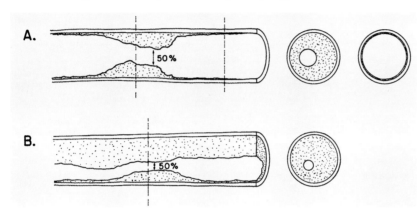

Fig. 11.8 Assessment of luminal narrowing. (a) The degree of luminal area occupied by a single stenotic lesion in an otherwise normal vessel is reasonably accurate, while **(b)** the estimated 50% of luminal narrowing of a severely diseased vessel markedly underestimates the amount of associated disease.

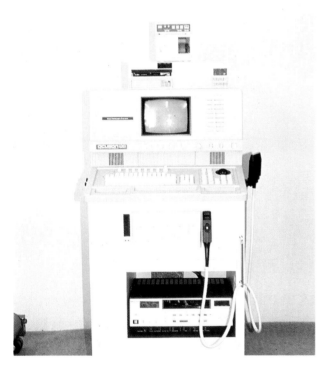

Fig. 11.9 Computerized, colour-coded duplex ultrasound machine. This is used for non-invasive imaging of the arterial or venous systems. (Courtesy of Dr J P Harris and Jenny Kidd, R N, Camperdown Vascular Laboratory, Sydney, Australia.)

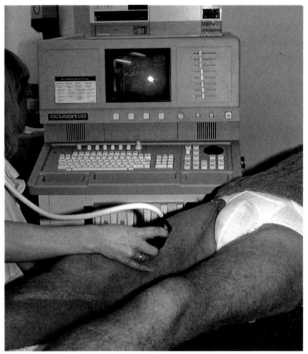

Fig. 11.10 Technique of ultrasound imaging with the probe held over the superficial femoral artery. (Courtesy of Dr J P Harris and Jenny Kidd, R N, Camperdown Vascular Laboratory, Sydney, Australia.)

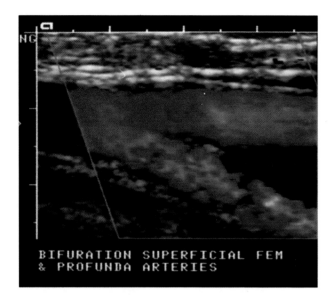

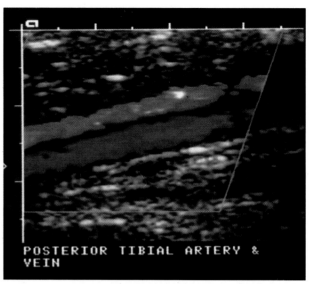

Fig. 11.11 Normal image of the bifurcation of the common femoral artery to the superficial and profunda femoris arteries. The homogeneous colour image represents normal, non-turbulent flow. (Courtesy of Dr J P Harris and Jenny Kidd, R N, Camperdown Vascular Laboratory, Sydney, Australia.)

Fig. 11.12 Normal image of the posterior tibial artery and vein. Forward flow in the artery is computer-coded red, while the reversed flow of blood in the vein is coded blue. (Courtesy of Dr J P Harris and Jenny Kidd, R N, Camperdown Vascular Laboratory, Sydney, Australia.)

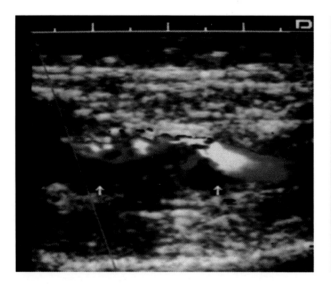

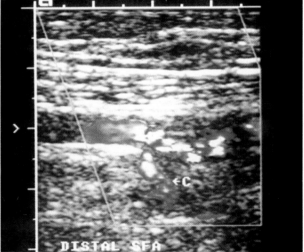

Fig. 11.13 A stenotic lesion of the superficial femoral artery, shown with heterogeneous colour break up in the region of turbulent flow. The limits of the stenosing plaque are indicated by the two arrows. (Courtesy of Dr J P Harris and Jenny Kidd, R N, Camperdown Vascular Laboratory, Sydney, Australia.)

Fig. 11.14 A tight stenosis of the superficial femoral artery, represented by the region of distorted, multicoloured, turbulent flow. The regions colour-coded blue represent reversal of arterial flow, indicative of severe stenosis. A collateral arterial branch is demonstrated immediately proximal to the stenotic lesion (C). (Courtesy of Dr J P Harris and Jenny Kidd, R N, Camperdown Vascular Laboratory, Sydney, Australia.)

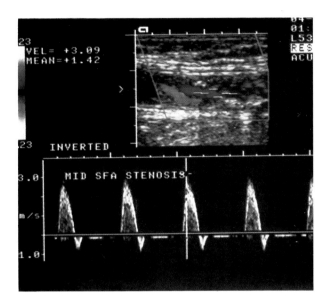

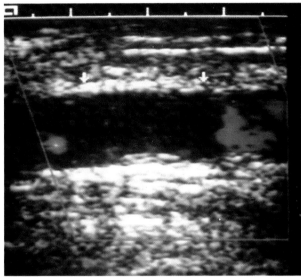

Fig. 11.15 Further information regarding a stenotic lesion may be derived from the waveform of the emitted sound spectrum. The height of the systolic wave is indicative of the velocity of flow through the lesion, and the waveform characteristics can also be used to quantify the degree of stenosis. (Courtesy of Dr J P Harris and Jenny Kidd, R N, Camperdown Vascular Laboratory, Sydney, Australia.)

Fig. 11.16 Total occlusion of the common femoral artery. This is indicated by the abrupt cessation of colour flow, and the ultrasonic echo shadows deep into the vessel. (Courtesy of Dr J P Harris and Jenny Kidd, R N, Camperdown Vascular Laboratory, Sydney, Australia.)

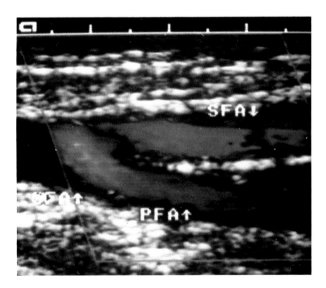

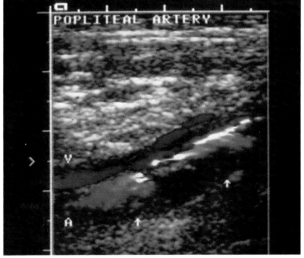

Fig. 11.17 Same patient as in Fig. 11.16; the image of the patent superficial femoral artery shows normal flow, being supplied by retrograde flow (blue) from the profunda femoris artery. (Courtesy of Dr J P Harris and Jenny Kidd, R N, Camperdown Vascular Laboratory, Sydney, Australia.)

Fig. 11.18 Colour flow image of a popliteal artery which has an adventitial cyst. Turbulent flow in the region of vessel distortion is shown. (Courtesy of Dr J P Harris and Jenny Kidd, R N, Camperdown, Vascular Laboratory, Sydney, Australia.)

INTRAVASCULAR ULTRASOUND

Intracardiac ultrasound catheters were first developed in 1956. Over the following two decades, improved delineation of intracardiac dimensions and cardiac images took place, resulting in better quality devices.

Recent advances in the catheter technology have led to intravascular ultrasound devices which generate images of the transmural anatomy of blood vessels, using 20–50 MHz transducers incorporated into the tip of the catheter. Although higher frequency has a limited tissue penetration, it is adequate for producing images when used intraluminally. At 20 MHz, the usable depth of penetration in blood is approximately 2–4 cm^3. At 50 MHz, the image resolution is finer, but penetration is more limited.

Ultrasound images are generated from piezoelectric transducers, by mechanically rotating an echotransducer or a mirror at the tip of a catheter, or by scanning with an array of stationary elements (Fig. 11.19).

The rotating intraluminal devices are simpler to manufacture, but the rotating transducer prototypes are more difficult to use in tortuous vessels, due to the necessity for rotating connection wires. This disadvantage is eliminated by the rotating mirror design or the multielement phase array configurations, although the increased electronic connection required in phase array devices

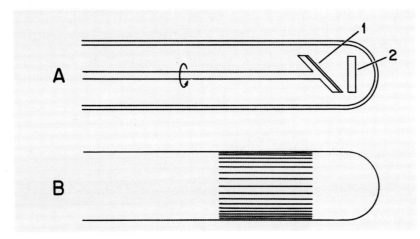

Fig. 11.19 (A) Prototype mechanical ultrasound device with (1) rotating and (2) fixed elements. Schematic representation. Either the transducer or the mirror may be fixed with the other element in a rotating position. **(B) Phased array device**, with the elements arranged circumferentially around the tip of the catheter. (From White, with permission; in press.)

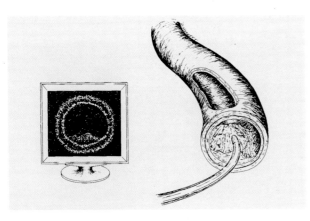

Fig. 11.20 Side viewing ultrasound device in an artery with a posterior wall plaque. Schematic representation. The image is obtained in a plane perpendicular to the vessel wall. (From White, with permission; in press.)

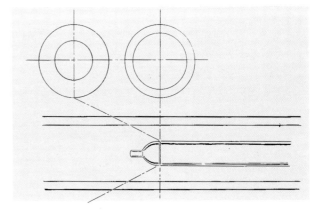

Fig. 11.21 Ultrasound probe within the lumen of a vessel. Schematic representation. Images obtained from a plane perpendicular to the device accurately display the vessel morphology, while wall thickness and location of lesions may be difficult to interpret in front viewing devices.

is difficult to miniaturize. Integrated circuits at the catheter tip may permit sequenced transmission; at the same time, these can improve flexibility and simplify manufacturing by reducing the number of wires in the catheter.

Ultrasound images produced by side viewing devices display the transmural anatomy of the arterial wall (Fig. 11.20). Potential forward viewing catheters are being developed, although the interpretation of wall thickness and lesion location are complicated by images obtained in a plane which is not perpendicular to the vessel wall (Fig. 11.21).

Clinical application of intraluminal ultrasound devices is easily accomplished in any procedure

where introduction of a 5–9F catheter is possible. Catheters as small as 3F are also being evaluated. Several prototype catheters can be passed over a guidewire, which enhances central positioning and imaging with the device (Fig. 11.22).

Images produced by intravascular ultrasound devices outline the luminal and adventitial surfaces of normal or minimally diseased arterial segments, with up to 0.1 mm accuracy (Fig. 11.23). Determination of the outside diameter of vessels is less accurate, with a margin error of up to 0.5 mm (Fig. 11.24).

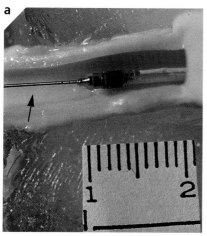
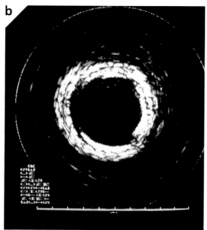

Fig. 11.22 (a) Phased array ultrasound probe (arrow) on the tip of a 5.5F catheter positioned in the lumen of an artery. A 0.14″ guidewire through a central lumen in the catheter helps to align the transducers perpendicular to the vessel wall. The artery is embedded in a silicone rubber mould for in vitro study of representative images. (b) Image of this vessel. (From Kopchok et al., 1990, with permission.)

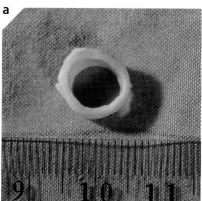
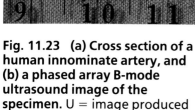
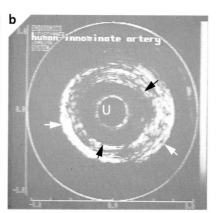
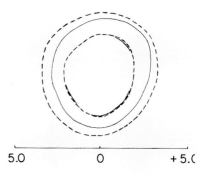

Fig. 11.23 (a) Cross section of a human innominate artery, and (b) a phased array B-mode ultrasound image of the specimen. U = image produced by ultrasound transducer; black arrows = intraluminal surface; white arrows = adventitial surface. (From White and White, 1989, with permission.)

Fig. 11.24 Correlation of inside and outside diameters of porcine vessels, measured by intravascular ultrasound (dotted lines), to those obtained by measured dimensions of the vessels (solid lines). (From Kopchok et al., 1990, with permission.)

Preliminary experimental and clinical studies using intravascular ultrasound catheters have demonstrated the ability of the devices to identify intraluminal thrombus, intimal flaps and artery wall dissections. Combined angioscopy and intraluminal ultrasound can also be used to delineate both luminal and transmural vessel wall anatomy (Figs 11.25 and 11.26).

Intravascular ultrasound provides a precise delineation of the vascular walls in vitro (see Figs 11.22 and 11.23), while in vivo evaluations may be more difficult to interpret (see Figs 11.25 and 11.26). As the technology improves, distinguishing vessel wall structures will be made easier. In muscular arteries, distinct layers of vessel wall may be visible, with the lumen and adventitia being more echogenic than the media (Fig.

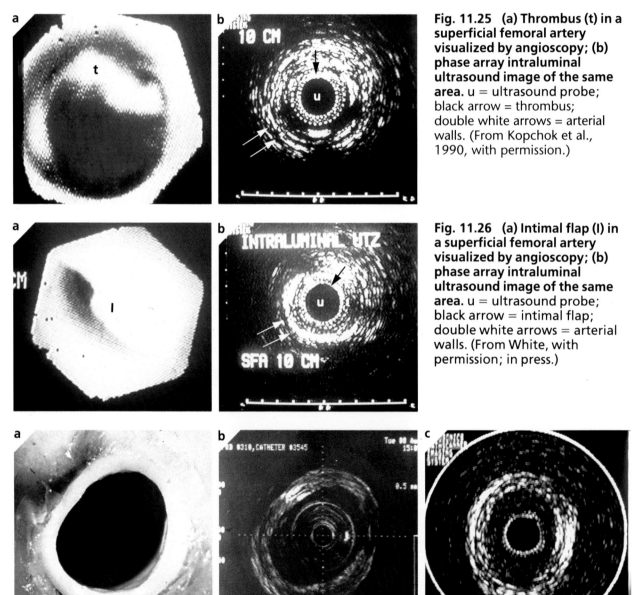

Fig. 11.25 (a) Thrombus (t) in a superficial femoral artery visualized by angioscopy; (b) phase array intraluminal ultrasound image of the same area. u = ultrasound probe; black arrow = thrombus; double white arrows = arterial walls. (From Kopchok et al., 1990, with permission.)

Fig. 11.26 (a) Intimal flap (I) in a superficial femoral artery visualized by angioscopy; (b) phase array intraluminal ultrasound image of the same area. u = ultrasound probe; black arrow = intimal flap; double white arrows = arterial walls. (From White, with permission; in press.)

Fig. 11.27 Human muscular artery embedded in silicone rubber mould (a); rotating intraluminal ultrasound image of the preparation (b). Three distinct layers corresponding to intima, media and adventitia of the vessel wall are apparent. Phase array intraluminal ultrasound image (c) of the same vessel seen in (a).

11.27b,c; these two views. also compare the images obtained from the rotating A-scan and phase array devices.

Small intimal lesions are quite well defined in muscular arteries, because of the fibrous tissue content (Fig. 11.28).

Four basic types of plaque contours can be distinguished by in vitro intravascular ultrasound imaging of human atherosclerotic arteries, using a 40 MHz rotating scan system. Hypoechoic images denote a significant deposit of lipid. Soft echoes reflect fibromuscular tissue (intimal proliferation), as well as lesions consisting of fibromuscular tissue and diffusely dispersed lipid. Bright echoes denote collagen-rich, fibrous tissue, and bright echoes with shadowing behind the lesion represent calcium (Fig. 11.29).

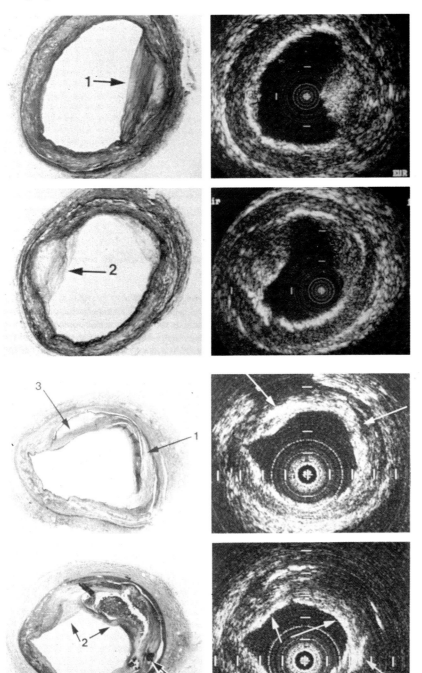

Fig. 11.28 Histological cross sections and ultrasound from a superior mesenteric artery. The media of this muscular artery, mainly composed of smooth cells, appears hypoechoic on ultrasound. Note that the eccentric atherosclerotic lesion, barely visible at the '9 o'clock' position, is of a markedly larger size compared to the cross section obtained 4 mm distally (lower pannel). Tissue from both lesions (arrows 1 and 2) was amorphous and non-calcific, containing fibromuscular tissue and lipid. Bright echoes of intima and adventitia circumscribe the hypoechoic media. Verhoeff van Giessen stain, × 8. (From Guessenhaven, Essel, Frietman et al., 1989, with permission.)

Fig. 11.29 Histological cross sections of a femoral artery. Fatty debris appearing as hypoechoic (arrow 1), collagen as bright echoes (arrow 2) and calcium as bright echoes with shadowing (arrow 3), are the major plaque constituents. Distribution of calcium within the lesion varies significantly ('11 o'clock' in the upper panel; '4 o'clock' in the lower pannel.) Upper pannel staining: Verhoeff van Giessen; lower pannel staining: Haematoxylin azophloxin. × 8. (From Guessenhaven, Essel, Frietman et al.,1989, with permission.)

Current limitations and future prospects

At present, and under optimal conditions, most ultrasound devices produce clear images of vessel anatomy. Careful positioning of catheter tips, and appropriate size ratios of probe to vessel, are required to optimize visualization in clinical situations. Image quality is best when the catheter is perpendicular to the wall, while minor angulations may affect image quality.

Eccentric positioning makes the near wall appear thicker and more echogenic. Methods to precisely identify the location and orientation of the probes are also required. With further development of these instruments, the current limitations related to image resolution and position sensitivity will be resolved.

Intraluminal vascular ultrasound is extremely promising in improving the guidance of angioplasty devices. The potential of intravascular ultrasound compared to other available guidance methods are illustrated in Table 11.1. This also stresses that ultrasound is the only method available which offers information on transmural wall architecture.

Table 11.1 Angioplasty Guidance				
	Luminal Morphology	Characterization	Vessel Wall Dimensions	Runoff
Fluoroscopy	+	–	–	+
Angioscopy	+	–/+	–	–/+
Spectroscopy	–	+	–	–
Ultrasound	+	+/–	+	–

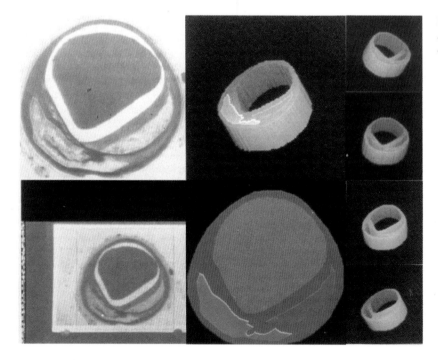

Fig. 11.30 Voxel model of an arterial section from a sequence of pathological slices. (From Kitney, Moura and Straughan, 1989, with permission.)

Future angioplasty guidance devices may combine the benefits of each modality in disposable delivery systems. Thus, visual inspection of the lumen by angioscopy, spectroscopy characterization of the tissue elements, and ultrasonic determination of the vessel wall and lesion dimensions would be possible. Improved intraluminal ultrasound devices will not only provide improved visualization of cross sectional vessel wall anatomy, but also a three-dimensional longitudinal reconstruction of the vasculature from a sequence of ultrasound images (Figs 11.30 and 11.31).

Colour doppler imaging may have additional applications in evaluating blood flow near vascular lesions.

The three-dimensional guidance of angioplasty catheters using intravascular ultrasound will help to eliminate the primary causes of failure of recanalizations and recurrence of lesions, as well as vessel wall perforation and inadequate debulking of lesions. The benefit which can be derived by concentric recanalization of occlusions, and the potential for perforation that exists in eccentric lesions, are illustrated in Fig. 11.32.

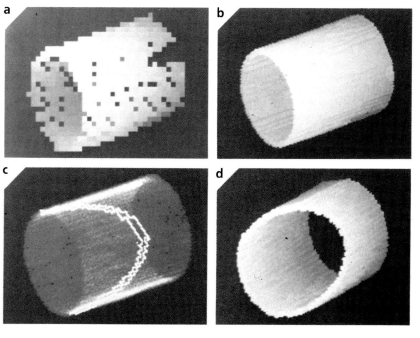

Fig. 11.31 Three-dimensional reconstruction of a section of a normal femoral artery from ultrasound data, recorded in vivo. (a) Low resolution model, used for rapid rotation. **(b)** Full resolution version of (a). **(c)** Transparent mode of (a), showing the contours of a potential oblique cut. **(d)** Full resolution version of (c). (From Kitney, Moura and Straughan, 1989, with permission.)

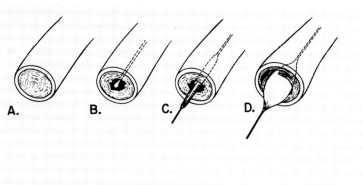

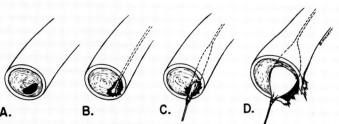

Fig. 11.32 Favourable outcome of concentric lesions (top), and enhanced potential for perforation of eccentric lesions (bottom) in currently used, balloon-assisted, angioplasty procedures. (From White and White, 1989, with permission.)

The discrepancy between the amount of debulking of lesions by current devices and methods of evaluation of repairs is emphasized in Fig. 11.33. The frequency of the incidence of inadequate debulking of lesions, leading to early thrombotic reocclusion or restenosis, remains undetermined. The importance of adequate removal of an atherosclerotic lesion, and the appropriate amount of material which should be removed to optimally delay the recurrence of stenosis, can only be assessed by a method like intravascular ultrasound, which defines with accuracy the vessel wall thickness and anatomical location of obstructions.

Using angioplasty catheters, which are used to perform vessel recanalizations and tissue removal guided by intravascular ultrasound, concentric debulking of lesions will be possible. This advance is required as a first step towards solving the limitations of current technology, related to inaccurate guidance of devices and inadequate tissue removal (Fig. 11.34).

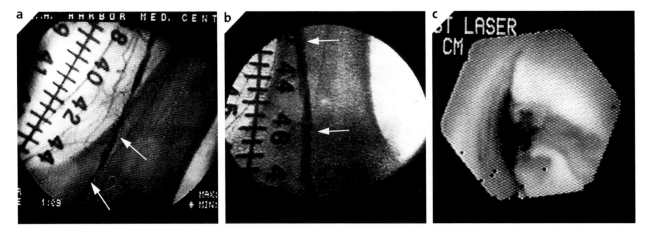

Fig. 11.33 (a) Fluoroscopic image of a superficial femoral artery lesion (white arrows); (b) same artery following laser-assisted balloon angioplasty, visualized with angiography, and (c) by angioscopy. Note the residual intraluminal material demonstrated by angioscopy, compared with a satisfactory result seen on radiography. (From White and White, 1989, with permission.)

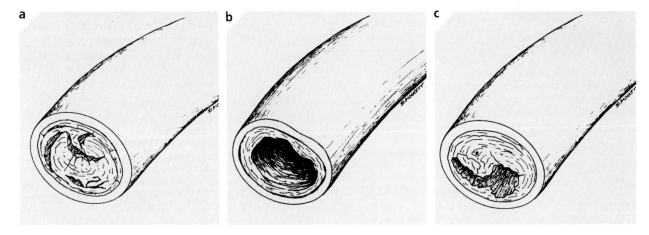

Fig. 11.34 (a) Arterial occlusion and (b) idealized, concentric recanalization. The latter can be accomplished by an intravascular ultrasound-guided device, compared to **(c)** which represents the limited success achieved by current methods.

References

Blackshear, W.M. and Strandness, D.E. (1981) Angiographic Imaging by Ultrasound Compared with Direct Methods, in *Investigation of Vascular Disorders* (eds A.N. Nicolaides and J.S.T Yao), Churchill Livingston, London, pp. 165–200.

Cieszynski, T. (1960) Intracardiac method for investigation of structure of the heart with the aid of ultrasonics, *Arch. Innun. Ter. Dow.*, 8, 551–7.

Coronary and Peripheral Angiography and Angioplasty (1989) (eds D.R. Leachman and R.D. Leachman), Edward Arnold, Division of Hodder and Stoughton, London.

Gussenhaven, W.J., Essel, C.E., Frietman, P., Mastik, F., Lancec, C., Slager, C., Serrvys, P., Gerriston, P., Pieterman, H. and Bom, H. (1989) Intravascular echographic assessment of vessel wall characteristics: a correlation with histology, *Int. J. of Cardiac Imag.*, 4, 105–16.

Interventional Cardiology and Angiology (1989) (eds B. Holfling and A. Polnitz), Springer–Verlag, New York, NY.

Intravascular Ultrasound: techniques, developments, clinical perspectives (1989) (eds N. Bom and J. Roelandt), Kluwer Academic Publishers, Dordrecht, The Netherlands.

Kitney R.I., Moura L. and Straughan K. (1989) 3-D visualization of arterial structures using ultrasound and voxel modelling. *Int. J. of Cardiac Imaging* 4, 135–43.

Kopckock G.E. *et al.* Intraluminal Ultrasound: A New Potential Modality for Angioplasty Guidance, Vascular Surgery, in press.

Kopckock G.E. *et al.* Intraluminal vascular ultrasound: Preliminary report of dimensional and morphologic accuracy. *Ann. Vasc. Surg.*, in press.

Lewis, B.D., James, M. and Welch, T.J. (1989) Current applications of duplex and color doppler ultrasound imaging: Carotid and peripheral vascular system. *Mayo. Clin. Proc.*, 64, 1147–57.

Sumner, D.S. (1982) Ultrasound in *Practical Noninvasive Vascular Diagnosis* (eds R.F. Kempezinski and J.S.T. Yao), Year Book Medical Publishers, Inc., Chicago, pp. 21–47.

Sumner D.S., Russell J.B., Miles R.D. (1983) Pulsed Doppler arteriography and computer assisted imaging of the carotid bifurcation, in *Cerebrovasular Insufficiency* (eds Bergan J.J. and Yao J.S.T.) Grune & Stratton, New York, NY, pp. 115–35.

Thiele, B.L. and Strandness, D.E. (1982) *Ultrasound Imaging In The Detection Of Carotid Disease* (eds R.E. Kompezinski and J.S.T. Yao), Year Book Medical Publishers, Inc., Chicago, pp. 239–61.

West, A.L. (1989) Endovascular ultrasound, in *Endovascular Surgery* (eds W.S. Moore and S.S. Ahn), WB Saunders Company, Philadelphia, Pennsylvania, pp. 518–23.

White, G.H., White, R.A. and Kopchok, G.E. (1989) Ancillary Modalities for endovascular surgery: Guidance systems, vascular stents, and methods to prevent restenosis, *Seminars In Vascular Surgery*, 2, 179–87.

White, R.A. Intravascular Ultrasound, in *Current Practice of Interventional Radiology* (eds S. Kadir and B.C. Decker), Inc., Philadelphia, PA, in press.

White, R.A., Kópchok, G.E., Hsiang, Y., Guthrie, C., Colman, P.D., Rosenbaum, D. and White, G. (1989) Perspectives for development of angioplasty guidance systems in Laser, in *Cardiovascular Disease* (eds R.A. White and W.S. Grundfest), Year Book Medical Publishers, Inc., Chicago, pp. 207–15.

White R.A. Indications for Fiberoptic Angioscopy and Intraluminal Ultrasound, Comprehensive Therapy, in press.

White R.A. Intravasular Ultrasound, in *Current Practice of Interventional Radiology* (ed. Kadir S.) B.C. Decker, Inc., Philadelphia, PA, in press.

White R.A. and White G.H. (1989) Laser Angioplasty: Development, current status, and future perspectives. *Seminars In Vascular Surgery*, 2, 123–42.

White R.A. and White G.H. (1989) Laser thermal probe recanalization of occluded arteries. *J. Vasc. Surg.* 9, 598–608.

12 Evolving Technology

VASCULAR TISSUE FUSION BY LASER

Tissue fusion by laser energy is an intriguing and very promising new development in laser technology. This method is particularly appealing for vascular procedures, for making sutureless blood vessel anastomoses, and for securing the endpoints of endarterectomies and dissection planes. Although there have been limited evaluations of this technology, preliminary experimental and clinical data are very promising for continued development and application.

In comparison to using high energy laser energy to ablate tissue as, for example, in angioplasty, soft tissue fusion is possible by delivering appropriate low levels of energy to the opposite tissue surfaces. The theoretical interactions of varying laser parameters in laser-tissue interactions, i.e. total energy delivered, pulse duration versus continuous wave delivery and concomitant thermal changes, are shown in Fig. 12.1.

In general, the higher energy applications ($> 100 \text{ J/cm}^2$, $> 100° \text{C}$) produce tissue ablation by optical means if the pulses are very short, and continuous wave lasers accomplish thermal ablation. At energy levels below the thermal vapourization range using normal pulse or continuous wave devices, the zone of thermal coagulation

and/or more likely lower temperature-reversible effects encompass the phenomenon occurring during tissue fusion.

Vascular tissue fusion or welding by lasers is performed by directing low power laser energy at the opposed edges of the repair. Several different wavelengths of energy, i.e. argon (515 nm), diode (830 nm), Nd : YAG (1060 and 1320 nm), holmium (2150 nm) and carbon dioxide (10 600 nm), have been evaluated for this application (Fig. 12.2).

The method of vessel wall apposition, aligning the tissue edges for application of laser energy, is shown in Fig. 12.3. Laser energy is applied to the vessel edges by moving the beam back and forth along the fusion line or, in certain cases, by delivering the energy through 'spot' delivery. The technique of laser welded vein to artery anastomosis is demonstrated in Fig. 12.4.

Vessel sealing is apparent to the trained eye in the majority of instances, as is non-union caused by inadequate energy delivery, or tissue coagulation or vapourization from excessive exposure (Fig. 12.5). Laser repairs can be undertaken in time intervals comparable to or slightly longer than those required for suture repairs.

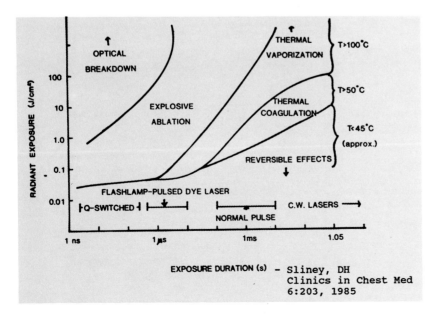

Fig. 12.1 Laser-tissue interactions. Biological effects depend on the duration of exposure. There are variable tissue temperatures for these effects; values and dividing lines are very approximate. (From Sliney, 1985, with permission.)

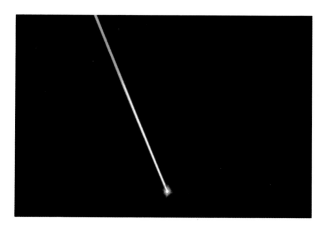

Fig. 12.2 Argon laser energy emitted from an optic fibre. This demonstrates the precise delivery of energy used at the site of tissue fusion.

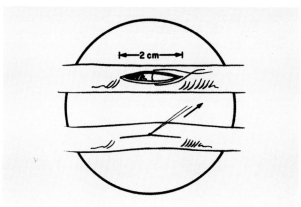

Fig. 12.3 Technique of laser welding of vessels, by aligning the tissue edges with traction sutures. (From White et al., 1985, with permission.)

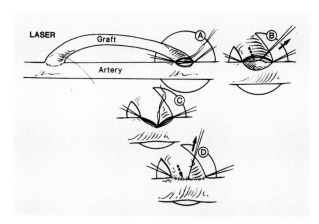

Fig. 12.4 Laser welding of the distal anastomosis of a vein bypass in the femoral artery. (a) Sutures are placed at the apices of incisions, and in the middle of the posterior wall. **(b)** Tension of the suture (solid arrow) in the middle of the posterior wall opposes the edges of repair for welding. A suture is placed in the middle of the anterior wall **(c)**, and opposes the edges for welding **(d)**. Broken arrow = site of laser energy delivery. (From White et al., 1988, with permission.)

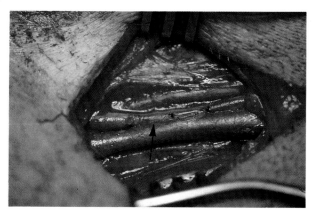

Fig. 12.5 Arteriovenous fistula immediately following argon laser fusion. Arrow marks the line of laser fusion between traction sutures placed at 1 cm intervals. (From White et al., 1988, with permission.)

Preliminary animal evaluations of laser fusion have demonstrated the ability to make vessel anastomoses which heal in the same way as control sutured specimens. However, the advantage of laser fusion is that reaction to the foreign body, persistent in wounds sutured with permanent materials, is eliminated (Fig. 12.6).

The adaptability of laser tissue fusion, both to microvessels and larger diameter (3–8 mm) veins and arteries, has been reported and successfully reproduced by many investigators. Different groups of investigators have their own preferences regarding the choice of laser, and it has to be established whether one or multiple wavelengths provide optimal fusions.

The mechanism of tissue fusions remains undetermined, and is probably laser-dependent. Lasers which cause significant heating of the tissues form

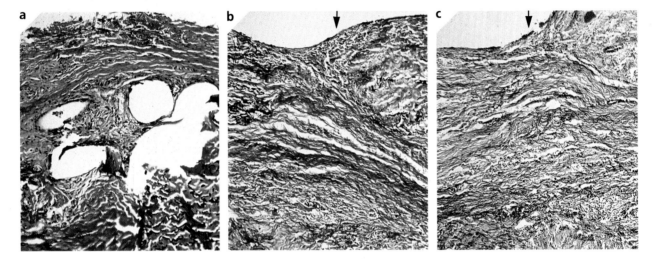

Fig. 12.6 Sutured and welded specimens. (a & b) Venotomies sutured and Nd: YAG laser welded five weeks previously. **(c)** A trichrome stain of the laser welded vein specimen. Laser welds **(b & c)** had near-normal vein architecture at the line of fusion (arrows), while sutured wounds **(a)** showed granulomatous reaction around the sutures, areas of excessive collagen accumulation and a broad gap in elastin continuity. The trichrome stain highlights the realignment of collagen fibres in the healed wound. Verhoeff van Giessen, × 10. (From White et al., 1986, with permission.)

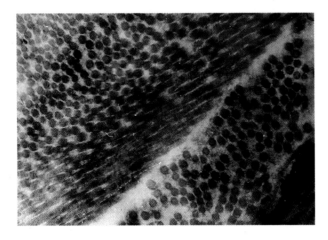

Fig. 12.7 Electron micrograph of collagen binding in areas of laser fusion. × 17 400. (From White et al., 1986, with permission.)

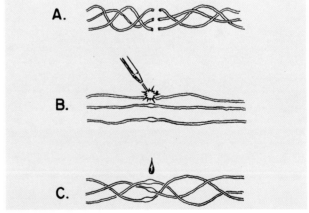

Fig. 12.8 (a) Apposition of collagen fibre in a tissue incision. **(b)** Mild heating of the collagen fibres by laser energy causes unwinding of the helical configuration. **(c)** Covalent bonds are formed in the annealing tissues, with cooling of the site by saline irrigation. (From White, with permission; in press.)

fusion primarily by adhesion of coagulated tissue elements. Other lower temperature techniques appear to cause tissue fusion by producing a high strength (covalent) bond between reannelling collagen fibres and other extracellular components (Fig. 12.7). The concept of argon laser tissue fusion is illustrated in Fig. 12.8.

Potential utility of the technology of vascular tissue fusion is related to the possibly improved healing at anastomotic sites, in comparison to sutured repairs. Preliminary canine studies have demonstrated less intimal hyperplasia in laser fused anastomoses, compared to sutured sites. This suggests that laser fusion may help to eliminate failure of clinical artery-vein anastomoses, caused by intimal proliferation (Figs 12.9 and 12.10).

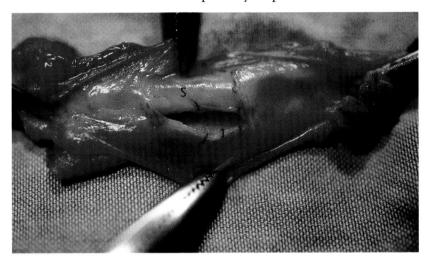

Fig. 12.9 Gross appearance of argon laser welded canine arteriovenous fistula, at eight weeks. S = traction sutures; 1 = 1 cm of laser fusion. (From White et al., 1987, with permission.)

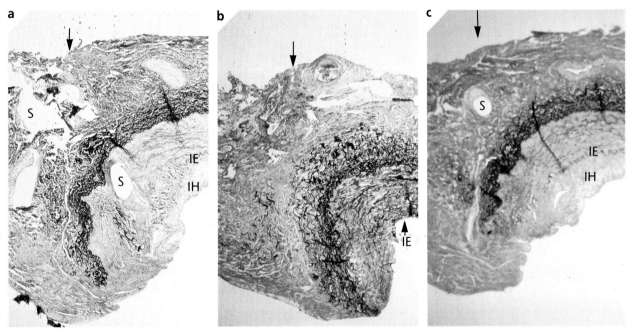

Fig. 12.10 (a) Sutured (a-v) fistulae at eight weeks; (b) argon laser sealed; (c) argon laser sealed at the site of a traction suture. Note that the sutured areas in control (a) and lasered specimen at the site of a traction suture (c) were associated with a marked intimal response. Arrows = line of artery-vein fusions; IE = internal elastic laminae; IH = intimal hyperplasia; S = suture holes. Verhoeff van Giessen, × 40. (From White et al., 1987, with permission.)

Initial human adaptability of argon laser fusion has been demonstrated, with successful healing and clinical performance of Cimino arteriovenous fistulas beyond a follow up of three years (Figs 12.11–12.15). Histological evaluation of tissue removed at the time of revision of two laser fused anastomoses, has demonstrated healing comparable to that found in the preclinical canine studies (Figs 12.16 and 12.17).

Research in animals and humans has evaluated the replacement of non-resorbable traction sutures with biodegradable sutures. The combination of laser fusion and biodegradable suturing is appealing, as the latter provides alignment of vessels during fusions and ensures initial strength until healing occurs. Subsequent resorption of the sutures prevents long term tissue reactions to the foreign body at the anastomotic line.

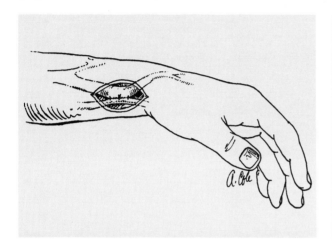

Fig. 12.11 **Initial trials of laser fusion of vascular tissue used human Cimino fistulas, constructed by connecting the brachial artery and cephalic vein in the forearm.** (From White, with permission; in press.)

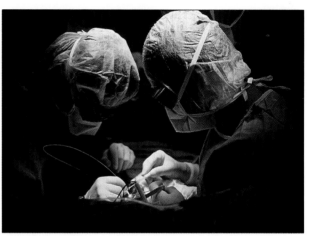

Fig. 12.12 **Argon laser light (blue), being delivered via an optic fibre to the anastomotic site.** Note the protective eyewear worn by the surgeons, to prevent eye damage from argon laser energy.

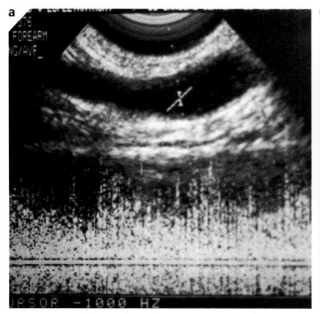

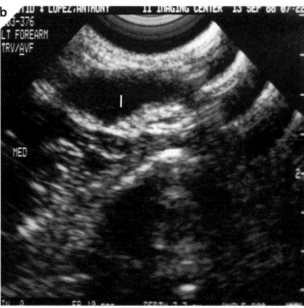

Fig. 12.13 **Duplex scan in longitudinal (a) and cross section (b) projections of a laser fused fistula, at two years following surgery.**

White line = line of anastomosis. (From White, with permission; in press.)

Initial evaluation of this method in humans and dogs has demonstrated healing of anastomoses, without luminal abnormality or aneurysm formation. Further development of this concept may eliminate the need for non-resorbable sutures in vessel anastomoses, and possibly improve the long term function of repairs.

Additional trials are being conducted to determine clinical adaptability of laser fusion of vascular tissue in humans, by applying it to form end-to-side artery-vein anastomoses in leg bypass procedures. The anastomotic technique is similar to that shown in Fig. 12.4. These trials will evaluate the utility of this technique in delaying or preventing anastomotic intimal complications; if a benefit is shown, then further clinical development and application may be justified.

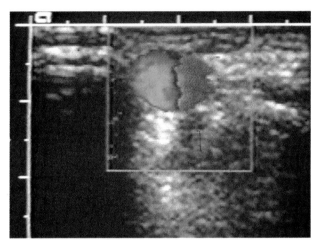

Fig. 12.14 Colour duplex of a second arteriovenous fistula, at two years following surgery. In this cross sectional view, the division of forward flow (towards the observer) in the artery (red), and return flow in the vein (blue), delineates the site of tissue fusion on the anterior (upper) and posterior (lower) walls of the fistula. Note the smooth transition at the fusion sites, with evidence of abnormal healing.

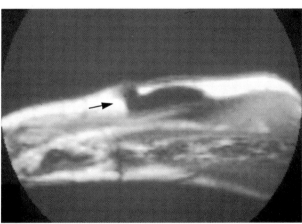

Fig. 12.15 Magnetic resonance imaging of laser fused arteriovenous fistulas, at five months following surgery. The transition from vein to artery at the site of anastomosis (arrow) is demonstrated. (From White et al., 1989, with permission.)

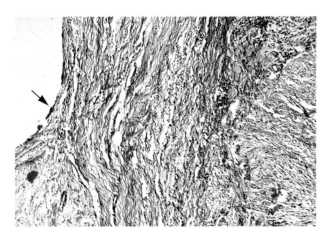

Fig. 12.16 Human laser fused arteriovenous fistula, at four months following surgery. The Cimino fistula was converted to a graft interposition, because of thrombosis of the proximal vein where dialysis was being performed. The laser fused segment showed regular orientation of the vascular wall architecture, and normal repair with no inflammation. Arrow = site of tissue fusion at the luminal surface. (From White, with permission; in press.)

Another intriguing use of the laser fusion technique has been in securing intimal endpoints of endarterectomies. This concept is quite appealing, as it addresses a problem which can be perplexing to the surgeon if the tissues are friable or inaccessible for conventional suture methods. Experimental evaluation has been extensive, and a limited number of trials in femoral and carotid artery endarterectomies have also been carried out in humans. The procedure combines endarterectomy performed by free laser energy, instead of a knife with laser fusion of the endarterectomy endpoints. This novel concept is demonstrated in Fig. 12.8.

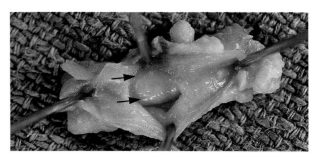

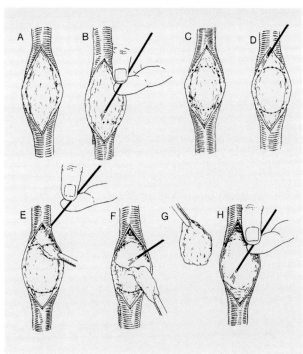

Fig. 12.17 Intraluminal appearance, ten months after surgery of a human arteriovenous fistula which was argon laser welded. Initially, the edges of anastomosis were opposed by biodegradable traction sutures at 0.5 mm intervals. The line of tissue fusion (arrow) demonstrates healing, with no evidence of remaining sutures. The specimen was retrieved at autopsy; the patient had died from an unrelated medical problem. (From White et al., with permission; in press.)

Fig. 12.18 (A) Arteriosclerotic artery opened longitudinally to expose an atheroma. (B) Lines of laser craters are created at one end of the atheroma, by individual laser exposures. **(C)** Individual laser exposures have been applied, to create lines of laser craters at both ends of the atheroma. **(D)** The lines of laser craters are connected by continuous laser radiation, to loosen the atheroma and create the sites for proximal and distal endpoints. **(E)** The atheroma is elevated away from the artery by continuous applications of laser light. **(F)** Continuous laser exposures are used, to develop the cleavage plane within the media and dissect the atheroma from the artery **(G)**. **(H)** The proximal and distal endpoints are welded by continuous laser radiation. (From Eugene, McColgan, Hammer-Wilson et al., 1985, with permission.)

References

Eugene, J., Baribeau, Y. and Berns, M.W. (1989) Laser endarterectomy, in *Lasers in Cardiovascular Disease* (eds R.A. White and W.S. Grundfest), Year Book Medical Publishers, Inc., Chicago, pp. 169–80.

Eugene, J., McColgan, S.J., Hammer-Wilson, M.E., *et al.* (1985) Laser endarterectomy. *Lasers Surg. Med.* 5, 265-74.

Murray, L.W., Su, L. Kopchok, G.E., Guthrie, C. and White R.A. (1989) Crosslinking of extracellular matrix proteins: A possible mechanism of argon laser welding. *Lasers Surg. Med.*, 9, 490–6.

Sliney D. (1985) Laser-tissue interactions. *Clinics In Chest Medicine* 6, 203-8.

White, R.A. Laser vascular tissue tusion: Development, Current Status and Future Perspectives. *J. Clin. Laser Med. Surg.*, in press.

White, R.A., Abergel, R.P., Lyons, R., Kopchok, G., Klein, S.R., Dwyer, R.M. and Uitto, J. (1986) Laser welding: An alternative method of venous repair. *J. Surg. Res.*, 41, 260–3.

White, R.A., Kopchok, G., Donayre, C., Lyons, R., White, G., Klein, S.R., Pizzurro, D., Abergel, R.P., Dwyer, R. and Uitto, J. (1987) Laser vessel sealing with the argon laser. *Lasers Surg. Med.*, 7, 229–35.

White, R.A., Kopchok, G.E., Donayre, C.E., Peng, S., Fujitani, R., White, G. and Uitto, J. (1988) Mechanism of tissue fusion in argon laser welded vein-artery anastomoses. *Lasers Surg. Med.*, 8, 83–9.

White, R.A., Kopchok, G., Donayre, C., White, G., Lyons, R., Abergel, R.P., Klein, S.R. and Uitto, J. (1987) Argon laser welded arteriovenous anastomosis, *J. Vasc. Surg.*, 6, 447–53.

White, R.A., Kopchok, G.E., Peng, S.K., Fujitani, R., White, G., Klein, S.R. and Uitto, J. (1987) Laser vascular welding—How does it work? *Ann. Vasc. Surg.*, 1, 461–4.

White, R.A., Kopchock, G.E., Vlasak, J., Hsiang, Y., Guthrie, C., Fujitani, R.M., White, G.H. and Peng, S.K. Experimental and early clinical evaluation of vascular anastomoses with argon laser fusion and the use of absorbable guy sutures: A preliminary report. *J. Vasc. Surg.*, in press.

White, R.A., Kopchok, G.E., White, G.H., Fujitani, R.M., Vlasak, J.W., Murray, L.W. and Peng, S.K. (1989) Laser-assisted vascular anastomoses, in *Lasers in Cardiovascular Disease* (eds R.A. White and W.S. Grundfest), Year Book Medical Publishers, Inc., Chicago, pp. 148–68.

White, R.A., White, G.H., Fujitani, R.M., Vlasak, J.W., Donayre, C.E., Kopchok, G.E. and Peng, S.K. (1989) Initial human evaluation of argon laser–assisted vascular anastomoses. *J. Vasc. Surg.*, 9, 542–7.

Index